Psychology and Sociology in Nursing

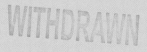

⑤SAGE | 50 YEARS

SAGE was founded in 1965 by Sara Miller McCune to support the dissemination of usable knowledge by publishing innovative and high-quality research and teaching content. Today, we publish more than 750 journals, including those of more than 300 learned societies, more than 800 new books per year, and a growing range of library products including archives, data, case studies, reports, conference highlights, and video. SAGE remains majority-owned by our founder, and after Sara's lifetime will become owned by a charitable trust that secures our continued independence.

Los Angeles | London | Washington DC | New Delhi | Singapore

2nd Edition

Psychology and Sociology in Nursing

Benny Goodman

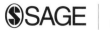

Los Angeles | London | New Delhi
Singapore | Washington DC | Boston

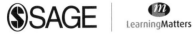

Learning Matters
An imprint of SAGE Publications Ltd
1 Oliver's Yard
55 City Road
London EC1Y 1SP

SAGE Publications Inc.
2455 Teller Road
Thousand Oaks, California 91320

SAGE Publications India Pvt Ltd
B 1/I 1 Mohan Cooperative Industrial Area
Mathura Road
New Delhi 110 044

SAGE Publications Asia-Pacific Pte Ltd
3 Church Street
#10-04 Samsung Hub
Singapore 049483

Commissioning editor: Alex Clabburn
Copy-editor: Liz Williams
Production controller: Chris Marke
Project management: Swales & Willis Ltd, Exeter,
Devon
Marketing manager: Camille Richmond
Cover design: Wendy Scott
Typeset by: C&M Digitals (P) Ltd, Chennai, India
Printed in Great Britain by CPI Group (UK) Ltd,
Croydon, CR0 4YY

Library of Congress Control Number: 2015930292

British Library Cataloguing in Publication data

A catalogue record for this book is available from
the British Library

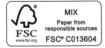

MIX
Paper from
responsible sources
FSC
www.fsc.org   FSC® C013604

ISBN 978-1-4739-1633-3
ISBN 978-1-4739-1634-0 (pbk)

At SAGE we take sustainability seriously. Most of our products are printed in the UK using FSC papers and boards.
When we print overseas we ensure sustainable papers are used as measured by the Egmont grading system.
We undertake an annual audit to monitor our sustainability.

Contents

Transforming Nursing Practice is a series tailor-made for pre-registration student nurses. Each book in the series is:

○ Affordable
○ Mapped to the NMC Standards and Essential Skills Clusters
○ Full of active learning features
○ Focused on applying theory to practice

Each book addresses a core topic and they have been carefully developed to be simple to use, quick to read and written in clear language.

"

An invaluable series of books that explicitly relates to the NMC standards. Each book cover a different topic that students need to explore in order to develop into a qualified nurse... I would recommend this series to all Pre-Registration nursing students whatever their field or year of study

Linda Robson
Senior Lecturer, Edge Hill University

The set of books is an excellent resource for students. The series is small, easily portable and valuable. I use the whole set on a regular basis.

Fiona Davies
Senior Nurse Lecturer, University of Derby

I recommend the SAGE/Learning Matters series to all my students as they are relevant and concise. Please keep up the good work.

Thomas Beary
Senior Lecturer in Mental Health Nursing, University of Hertfordshire

"

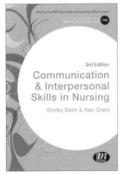

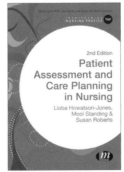

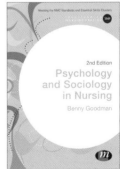

CORE KNOWLEDGE TITLES:

Becoming a Registered Nurse: Making the Transition to Practice

Communication and Interpersonal Skills in Nursing (3rd Ed)

Contexts of Contemporary Nursing (2nd Ed)

Getting into Nursing (2nd Ed)

Health Promotion and Public Health for Nursing Students (2nd Ed)

Introduction to Medicines Management in Nursing

Law and Professional Issues in Nursing (3rd Ed)

Leadership, Management and Team Working in Nursing (2nd Ed)

Learning Skills for Nursing Students

Medicines Management in Children's Nursing

Nursing and Collaborative Practice (2nd Ed)

Nursing and Mental Health Care

Nursing in Partnership with Patients and Carers

Passing Calculations Tests for Nursing Students (3rd Ed)

Palliative and End of Life Care in Nursing

Patient Assessment and Care Planning in Nursing (2nd Ed)

Patient and Carer Participation in Nursing

Patient Safety and Managing Risk in Nursing

Psychology and Sociology in Nursing (2nd Ed)

Successful Practice Learning for Nursing Students (2nd Ed)

Understanding Ethics in Nursing Practice

Using Health Policy in Nursing

What is Nursing? Exploring Theory and Practice (3rd Ed)

PERSONAL AND PROFESSIONAL LEARNING SKILLS TITLES:

Clinical Judgement and Decision Making for Nursing Students (2nd Ed)

Critical Thinking and Writing for Nursing Students (2nd Ed)

Evidence-based Practice in Nursing (2nd Ed)

Information Skills for Nursing Students

Reflective Practice in Nursing (2nd Ed)

Succeeding in Essays, Exams & OSCEs for Nursing Students

Succeeding in Literature Reviews and Research Project Plans for Nursing Students (2nd Ed)

Successful Professional Portfolios for Nursing Students (2nd Ed)

Understanding Research for Nursing Students (2nd Ed)

MENTAL HEALTH NURSING TITLES:

Assessment and Decision Making in Mental Health Nursing

Engagement and Therapeutic Communication in Mental Health Nursing

Medicines Management in Mental Health Nursing

Mental Health Law in Nursing

Physical Healthcare and Promotion in Mental Health Nursing

Psychosocial Interventions in Mental Health Nursing

ADULT NURSING TITLES:

Acute and Critical Care in Adult Nursing

Caring for Older People in Nursing

Medicines Management in Adult Nursing

Nursing Adults with Long Term Conditions

Safeguarding Adults in Nursing Practice

Dementia Care in Nursing

You can find more information on each of these titles and our other learning resources at **www.sagepub.co.uk**. Many of these titles are also available in various e-book formats, please visit our website for more information.

About the author

Benny Goodman, following an earlier career in the Royal Navy, graduated with a degree in Sociology and Politics in 1986, and has been a Lecturer in Adult Nursing at Plymouth University since 1992. His clinical focus has been adult acute hospital-based care, and new roles for nurse practitioners, paramedics and emergency care practitioners in health assessment and clinical examination. His developing research and teaching focus is on sociology and sustainability, climate change and health. He teaches courses that draw students from various disciplinary and professional backgrounds.

Introduction

Who is this book for?

This book is primarily for students of nursing who wish to progress on to the register. However, it may also be used by students on health studies and health and social care courses at NVQ, BTEC, Foundation degree and degree level. It should be relevant across all three years of a typical nursing degree. The focus is not to develop knowledge for any one specific 'field' of nursing (adult, child, mental health, learning disabilities) but to support development across all the fields. Although the Nursing and Midwifery Council's 2010 (NMC) standards are a foundation for what follows, the content is not narrowly defined by them.

Nursing, health, well-being and illness

Many students – and even qualified nurses – struggle to understand what the disciplines of psychology and sociology have to do with them. I believe these disciplines are fundamental for helping you to understand your patients (both as individuals and as part of the wider society) and indeed for developing your own professional practice. The aim in writing this book, therefore, is to help you understand the relevance and connectedness of psychology and sociology to your nursing practice. I want to help you use the knowledge offered by these disciplines to deepen the effectiveness of your interactions with, and care of, your patients.

Psychology and sociology are two of the social sciences. Science-based care (and evidence-based care) is foundational for nursing practice. An understanding of all the sciences, not just the physical sciences, will help you to become a more effective practitioner.

Before turning to the impact of psychological and sociological factors on health and well-being, it must be acknowledged that a great deal of work in the NHS focuses on illness and disease. This fact is reflected by the argument of Peter Morrall (2009) that medicine and nursing are primarily *disciplines of disease*. Disease produces physical, psychological and social responses and, from a sociological perspective, can have more to do with issues of social structure than biology. For example, at the physical level an infection will cause an immune response resulting in pyrexia, redness, swelling, pain and alteration of function in the infected part. At the psychological level there will be the individual's affective (feelings), cognitive (knowledge) and behavioural responses. One such response could be withdrawal from work responsibilities. At the sociological level there will be a social response to people who have infections. These responses could be fear, shame, avoidance or blame, which may lead to the stigmatising of a group (such as those with HIV infection). In addition to social response, there are social patterns to infection (and other diseases) that result in some people being more at risk than others to a significant degree because of their place in the social hierarchy.

> *The social determinants of health are the conditions in which people are born, grow, live, work and age,*
> *including the health system. These circumstances are shaped by the distribution of money, power and*
> *resources at global, national and local levels, which are themselves influenced by policy choices. The*
> *social determinants of health are mostly responsible for health inequities – the unfair and avoidable*
> *differences in health status seen within and between countries.*
> (World Health Organization, 2008)

Health and well-being, therefore, are founded upon a complex mix of biology and an individual's psychosocial existence. In addition to this is the social and political environment, which is addressed by the *social determinants of health* approach. Studies from both disciplines indicate that any understanding of health, and interventions to promote well-being, have to take into account the wider context in which individuals, groups, communities and populations live. One small example is the co-relationship between geography and life expectancy. Life expectancy at birth in the UK for 2006–2008 was highest in the south of England. Life expectancy was 79.2 years for males in the south-east and 83.1 years for females in the south-west. In contrast, Scotland had the lowest life expectancy at birth in the UK, at 75.0 years for males and 79.9 years for females (Office for National Statistics, 2009).

What is psychology?

Psychology is the science of mind and behaviour (Gross and Kinnison, 2013). The complexity of the human mind means that it is not simply explained and different theoretical perspectives have been used to study and understand our species. The perspectives used by psychologists can be grouped under three headings, each with a different focus on the human condition. Some psychologists focus on the emotional (or 'affective') aspect of humanity, studying how feelings influence our development and the way we view the world. Other psychologists adopt a cognitive approach and investigate thinking, memory and decision making. The third group use a behavioural approach and study observable human actions, responses to stimuli and how we learn our behaviours. The behaviourists are also referred to as learning theorists. While grouping the many psychological perspectives under three headings may help us understand the bias within the theory, many practising psychologists have an eclectic or inclusive view of people. It is important for nurses to acknowledge the role that affect, cognition and behaviour play in making their patients the individuals they are.

What is sociology?

According to the British Sociological Association (2010), sociology is the *study of how society is organized and how we experience life*. This definition has the benefit of being brief, but not too illuminating. Sharp (2010) argues that sociology is the study of *human society*, and thus its scope is almost limitless. Any human activity at individual (micro) level and at societal (macro) level could be the object of investigation, study and questioning. Typical subjects include the forms and functions of the family; the world of work and organisations; social class; ethnicity and gender relationships. The sociology of health and illness is an area of study that has its own journal, *Sociology of Health and Illness*, in which are published articles on all aspects of health, illness, medicine and healthcare.

As with psychology, a striking feature of sociology is the various viewpoints or 'perspectives' which the (very) different theorists use, both to ask questions and to answer them. For example, a feminist perspective might be interested in the place of women in society and how the medical profession 'controls' childbirth in hospitals. A Marxist perspective may address how medical professionals have focused for too long on the individual cause of disease at the expense of the *social determinants of health* (World Health Organization, 2008). It will be helpful for you as a nurse to gather an understanding of a variety of different sociological perspectives on aspects of healthcare.

Psychology, sociology and you

In the light of the information above, are you starting to get a glimpse of how psychology and sociology might impact on your everyday work as a nurse? If you are nursing adults, for example, you will not only be called upon to dress an infected wound; you will also need to have some understanding of what it means for an individual in our society to have a chronic wound. You may then find yourself needing to think about and address the social causes and policy implications of infections.

It is absolutely crucial for the mental health nurse to understand the various psychological and social theories that underpin the diagnosis, treatment and management of mental illness. In recent history in the UK, the transition of care in institutions to care in the community reflects such theoretical application from the social sciences. The use of drugs and of 'talking therapies' are both based on scientific notions of the nature and the cause of illness and health.

Children's nurses need to understand and deliver the care of children in the context of knowledge about family relationships as well as the psychological development that children may go through. Nurses caring for people with learning disabilities need to understand how society designs and delivers care for vulnerable adults. They also need to be aware of care theories such as social role valorisation.

A note on genetic factors

According to Professor Steve Jones (2009), the search for genetic causes for behaviour (i.e. finding a gene 'for' something) is misplaced. Scientists had embarked on a search for rogue genes responsible for just about every modern malady, hoping such conditions could be blamed on a small set of genes, which could then lead to a cure. But the more they investigated, the more complicated they realised it would be to find a cure. It is argued that many individual genes say very little about the real risk of disease, and scientists have found diet and the environment still have an enormous influence on whether we develop a disease.

Concept summary: Epigenetics

The term *epigenetics* refers to changes in phenotype (appearance) or gene expression caused by mechanisms other than changes in the underlying DNA sequence. This means environmental factors can affect genes, challenging the idea of genetic determination (a gene 'for' something). In addition, there is little or no mention of genetic factors being implicated in the development of poor mental health. The risk factors for mental illness in adults include unemployment, low income, debt, violence, stressful life events, inadequate housing, fuel poverty and other adversity (Royal College of Psychiatrists, 2010).

Requirements from the NMC standards

The process of nursing is based on a therapeutic relationship that requires the nurse to have particular skills. The NMC standards (2010) describe four knowledge domains to underpin these skills:

1. professional values;
2. communication and interpersonal skills;
3. nursing practice and decision making;
4. leadership, management and team working.

These standards are used by educational organisations when planning and designing their courses. The book will draw from all four domains and will present the relevant standards at the beginning of each chapter.

The standards also set out what the content of education provision should be. The most pertinent aspects of the standards for this book are:

From requirement 5.6.1:

- professional codes, ethics, law and humanities;
- health and behavioural sciences;
- principles of national and international health policy, including public health.

From requirement 5.6.2:

- communication, compassion and dignity;
- emotional support;
- equality, diversity, inclusiveness and rights;
- identity, appearance and self-worth;
- autonomy, independence and self-care;
- public health and promoting health and well-being.

From EU Directive 2005:

(a) adequate knowledge of the sciences on which general nursing is based, including sufficient understanding of the structure, physiological functions and behaviour of healthy and sick persons, and of the relationship between the state of health and the physical and social environment of the human being;
(b) sufficient knowledge of the nature and ethics of the profession and of the general principles of health and nursing.

Book structure

Chapter 1 looks at why psychology and sociology are relevant for nursing. A contemporary issue of national interest, the Mid Staffordshire NHS Foundation Trust Inquiry (Francis, 2010), is used to highlight many sociological and psychological issues relevant to nursing. These include issues such as occupational socialisation, obedience ('just following orders'), communications, effect from the individual nurse's decisions through to the macro-level reasons behind why the problems at Mid Staffordshire NHS Foundation Trusts happened. C. Wright Mills' (1959) ideas about the relationship between society and the individual are also explored.

Chapter 2 takes a critical look at the notion of professional values. Values can be discussed and listed, as has been done by the NMC. However, what professionals actually do needs critical examination. After all, the issues at Mid Staffs arose within a context of 'professional' practice. We need, therefore, to investigate what we mean by 'professional' and to consider how professions operate in society. We need to examine the professional–patient relationship and consider what is ethical professional practice. Finally, we have to revisit the meaning of 'care'.

Chapter 3 explores communication. We begin by examining the fundamentals of verbal and non-verbal communication before looking at ideas around perception and self. This is because communicating with others is based on how we perceive ourselves and how we perceive others. Goffman's (1963) notion of stigma is covered, along with labelling theory. Finally, the chapter looks briefly at how new communication technologies impact on nursing practice and the way we relate to patients.

Chapter 4 is concerned with nursing practice. In particular, it considers nursing practice as a *social activity* that takes place within the context of inequalities in health and the *social determinants of health approach* (World Health Organization, 2008). This balances the individual and biomedical focus of much of nursing practice, which is discussed in many other books.

Nurses are required to undertake practice and make decisions underpinned by the 'best available evidence', so Chapter 5 is concerned with decision making. Issues around what is accepted as evidence, and how evidence is accepted and used, are central, and complementary medicine is used as an example of this. International drug policy is used as an example of how evidence gets used and affected by policy decisions. In addition, the chapter looks at national and international guidelines, processes of decision making and the use of *errors in thinking*, heuristics and mental 'short cuts'.

Chapter 6 looks at leadership, which is examined in the wider context in which nurses in the UK NHS operate. It picks up the argument of Hewison and Griffiths that *although [leadership] is a key area for development, of equal, if not greater importance, is the need for NHS organisations to create the conditions which support and enhance new models of leadership* (2004, p. 471). The findings of the Mid Staffs enquiry are considered in this context. We attempt to examine the personal troubles that nurses and patients experience (e.g. low morale and poor quality care) in the context of the public issues (e.g. infection rates, abuse in Mid Staffs and elsewhere) and in terms of the structural transformations faced by society (e.g. reform(s) of NHS organisations, rising public expectations and increasing demands on services, ageing populations). This will help to put issues of leadership into some sort of social context, to understand more fully (and hopefully begin to deal with) the current and future (e.g. climate change) issues of our times.

Death will affect everyone, whether or not they work in healthcare, and Chapter 7 helps us to reflect on what this means both for ourselves and for our patients. We begin with an overview of the social nature of death before exploring it from a more individual and personal nature. Nurses will be better able to deal with the various understandings and meanings people attach to death and dying if they realise that dying is not a purely personal and biological event. An understanding of the social nature of death helps to challenge assumptions and taken-for-granted beliefs. The chapter goes on to discuss stress and coping with challenging events, and looks at ways to improve our well-being.

The NMC outlines fields for nursing practice and all nurses have to address fields other than their own. Chapters 8 and 9 outline some psychosocial issues in the fields of nursing that will be useful to student nurses who will need to provide evidence of achieving certain learning outcomes. Chapter 8 concentrates on maternity and child health, while Chapter 9 is concerned with the fields of mental health and learning disabilities as field/patient group-specific issues. This material relates to the European Union requirements for general care in each of these areas.

Finally, a brief conclusion will summarise and address current issues and future directions. We hope that this will stimulate some provocative thinking.

Learning features and activities

Learning from text is not easy. For some it may not feel like learning at all! Therefore to provide variety and to assist with the development of reflective and critical thought, this book contains reflective tasks, case studies and further reading to enable you to participate in your own learning. At various stages within each chapter there are points at which you can break to undertake activities. Undertaking and understanding the activities are important elements of your understanding of the content of each chapter. You are encouraged, where appropriate, to reflect on your practice and consider how the things you have learned from working with patients might inform your understanding of patient assessment and care planning. You will need to develop your own study skills, and 'learn how to learn' in order to get the best from the material. In particular, we encourage you to learn how to access and analyse material and to be literate with new digital media.

Other activities will require you to take time away from the book to find out new information which will add to your understanding of the ways in which psychology and sociological concepts impact upon healthcare, as well as the ways in which psychological and sociological understanding can improve your own practice and awareness. Some activities challenge you to apply your learning to a question or scenario to help you reflect on issues and practice in more depth. A few activities require you to make observations during your day-to-day life or in the clinical setting. In some cases, you are encouraged to discuss your thoughts or findings with a mentor or one or more fellow students. All the activities in this book are designed to increase your understanding of the topics under discussion and how they impact upon nursing practice.

Chapter 1
The relevance of psychology and sociology for nursing

NMC Standards for Pre-registration Nursing Education

This chapter will address the following competencies:

Domain 1: Professional values

1. All nurses must practise with confidence according to *The Code: Standards of Conduct, Performance and Ethics for Nurses and Midwives* (NMC, 2008), and within other recognised ethical and legal frameworks. They must be able to recognise and address ethical challenges relating to people's choices and decision-making about their care, and act within the law to help them and their families and carers find acceptable solutions.

2. All nurses must practise in a holistic, non-judgemental, caring and sensitive manner that avoids assumptions, supports social inclusion; recognises and respects individual choice; and acknowledges diversity. Where necessary, they must challenge inequality, discrimination and exclusion from access to care.

Domain 2: Communication and interpersonal skills

4. All nurses must recognise when people are anxious or in distress and respond effectively, using therapeutic principles, to promote their wellbeing, manage personal safety and resolve conflict. They must use effective communication strategies and negotiation techniques to achieve best outcomes, respecting the dignity and human rights of all concerned. They must know when to consult a third party and how to make referrals for advocacy, mediation or arbitration.

Domain 4: Leadership, management and team working

4. All nurses must be self-aware and recognise how their own values, principles and assumptions may affect their practice. They must maintain their own personal and professional development, learning from experience, through supervision, feedback, reflection and evaluation.

Chapter aims

After reading this chapter, you will be able to:

*   discuss the relevance of sociology and psychology to nursing;
*   outline some of the key ideas in sociology, such as the 'sociological imagination', and their relevance to nursing;

- outline some of the key ideas in psychology, such as 'obedience', and their relevance to nursing;
- appreciate how psychology and sociology are interlinked;
- discuss how this understanding applies to contemporary issues such as the Mid Staffordshire NHS Foundation Trust Inquiry.

Introduction

This chapter discusses why sociology and psychology are relevant for nursing practice. Following a brief description of the two sciences, we will examine the relevance of the *sociological imagination* (Wright Mills, 1959; Goodman, 2011a; Rolfe, 2011). Then, the Francis reports (Francis, 2010, 2013) into the failings at Mid Staffordshire NHS Trust will be used to illustrate some important psychological ideas such as obedience, moral disengagement, prejudice and the humanistic therapeutic relationship.

Sociology and psychology underpin many aspects of the nursing role and your interactions with individuals, communities and populations. This is why the Nursing and Midwifery Council (NMC) has specified that you must cover social and behavioural sciences. Some students struggle to see the relevance of sociology to their experience of nursing in clinical practice (Edgley et al., 2009), and there have been critiques (Sharp, 1994, 1995).

Sociology

Sociology is characterised by various perspectives (Haralambos and Holborn, 2013) and does not present one version of social life. Crudely, these perspectives are:

- functionalism;
- Marxism;
- feminism;
- interactionism;
- phenomenology;
- postmodernism.

You do not need an indepth understanding of these approaches, as you are not studying sociology. However you do need to understand that sociologists often see the social world in very different ways. Similarly, nursing is complex decision making involving critical self-reflection based on competing philosophies and theories, operating in power and social contexts, addressing populations as well as individuals. An argument is that the knowledge needed by nurses is not just for action in practical settings ('know how') but for personal and social transformation ('know why') and sociology might help in this regard.

Concept summary: The case for sociology in nursing

Mulholland (1997) maintains that sociology:

- provides an alternative to individualistic biomedical models;
- supports critical and self-reflective practice;
- addresses the exercise of power;
- encourages a *quality of mind* (Wright Mills, 1959);
- challenges the 'taken for granted';
- involves the 'know why', not just the 'know how'.

Although reflection is an important concept in nurse education and practice, you may find it difficult to achieve when you are starting out. However, concentrating on biomedically based nursing makes sociology seem difficult, which in turn can have a negative effect on our understanding of what nursing practice is (see, for example, Morrall, 2001).

To counter this, we need to see that the social sciences can help to demystify the subjective experience of illness and objective patterns of health and disease. This may also bring to the fore the social nature of disease and death, shining an analytical light on the power relationships involved and the ethical issues experienced. This will hopefully help to create a discerning nurse who becomes better at decision making. This is what Peter Morrall (2009) calls for as *moral action* to complement our understanding and our practice as clean, competent and kind nurses.

Sociology encourages and requires transformational learning, which does not sit easily within the current practical and power context of much of nursing practice. However, when you engage with the wider issues, understand that there are different ways of knowing and examine what it means to develop a sociological imagination (Wright Mills, 1959), an opportunity exists for you to develop into a *knowledgeable doer* (UKCC, 1986), able to transform yourself, your nursing practice and in turn society (Goodman, 2011a).

Psychology

One way to use psychology is to consider a psychological idea and apply it to a nurse's understanding about people and challenging a personal viewpoint. This requires reading around the topic area and identifying ideas that might have something to say about working with people. For example in the 'psychology of ageing' literature you may read about 'gerotranscendence' and 'disengagement theory'.

Tornstam (1997) discussed the idea of gerotranscendence, which suggests that growing old is part of normal development and can result in us progressing towards being more mature and wise. It is a positive view of ageing. If this is the case, the nurse should understand that age is not necessarily a negative experience and should accept that older people indeed have a degree of understanding about life that brings positive benefits. This theory, Tornstam suggests, is a counter to 'disengagement theory' (Cumming and Henry, 1961), in that the older person engages in new perspectives and understandings rather than withdrawing, or disengaging, from society.

Another idea is that of 'learned helplessness'.

Learned helplessness (Seligman, 1975) is a state of depression caused by perceived lack of control and may result in negative thinking, behaviour and motivation. Therefore a nurse may ensure that all possible decisions about patients and their care are not taken away, that patients remain in control of their activities of daily living. If this is not the case, if care professionals remove control, then patients may lapse into depression.

To help further, a search of the literature reveals the study described below.

Liu et al. (2012) undertook a systematic review of the literature to look at nurses' attitudes to older people. They suggest that attitudes were inconsistent and that since 2000 were perhaps less positive. The age, gender and education of the nurses were not predictors of their attitudes. This suggests that nurses' views on ideas such as gerotranscendence and control might be quite variable. Liu et al. state that *negative attitudes towards older people and myths about ageing are ubiquitous* (p. 1271). If this is the case, this supports the theories around negative *stereotyping* (Fiske and Taylor, 1991) and *prejudice* (Allport, 1954) that nurses might apply to older people. Therefore nurses need to reflect on their own stereotypes, attitudes and prejudices towards older people and, having done so, to behave towards them as human beings, not as 'old people'.

Just as there many perspectives in sociology (Haralambos and Holborn, 2013), psychology also has various perspectives (Walker et al., 2012):

- social psychology;
- behaviourism;
- humanistic psychology;
- cognitive psychology;
- psychodynamic.

In this section we will examine just a few to illustrate the differing approaches.

Activity 1.1 *Reflection*

How obedient are you?

If your mentor told you to leave a patient lying in a soiled bed because that patient needed to be taught a lesson, what would you do? How would you feel?

Can you identify a situation where you have gone along with a group decision despite feeling a little uneasy, either at the time or later on?

You do not need to share this reflection with anyone unless you want to.

As this activity is based on your personal thoughts and reflections, there is no sample answer at the end of the chapter.

Obedience

We can see several social psychological factors in operation in this activity: your role as a student; your mentor's role as a qualified nurse and the difference in your status.

We may like to think that our actions are always based on individual free will, clear moral codes and avoidance of actual harm. The social psychologist Stanley Milgram (1963) began a series of experiments to investigate what makes ordinary people perform 'barbaric' acts. He began by asking psychiatrists and psychologists what proportion of the population would give a fatal electric shock on the orders of another person. Most of the experts thought around 1 per cent of the population would perform such an act, but the results of Milgram's experiments were enlightening. Milgram found that 65 per cent of subjects would go all the way up to 450 volts.

Milgram's experiment caused much debate and triggered other experiments like that performed by Hofling et al. (1966). This study of obedience took place in the natural setting of a psychiatric hospital. Boxes of placebo tablets were placed on 22 wards. The containers were marked: Astrofen 5 mg, maximum daily dose 10 mg. The experimenter then rang the ward, saying that he was Dr Smith, and instructing the nurse who replied to give his patient, Mr Jones, 20 mg of Astrofen, as he was in a desperate hurry and the patient needed to have the tablets. He said that he would be there in 10 minutes to sign the prescription and see the patient. The observer on the ward noted that 21 out of 22 nurses went on to give the medication. The nurse who refused was a student.

Activity 1.2   *Research and evidence-based practice*

We do not like to think of ourselves as conforming and obedient. Use the internet to find out more about Milgram's experiment and the controversy it provoked. For example:

www.spring.org.uk/2007/02/stanley-milgram-obedience-to-authority.php

Who were the participants and what roles were they asked to play? What 'treatments' were applied?

What percentage of participants continued to apply the treatment despite the reactions they witnessed?

Describe a possible flaw in the experiment.

There are outline answers to this activity at the end of the chapter.

When the nurses in the Hofling study broke the rules for giving medication, they saw the person giving the order as responsible. They failed to see or remember that they should *never* give a drug with which they are unfamiliar. They also ignored the facts that the drug exceeded the stated safe dose, it was not prescribed and that verbal orders from unknown doctors are not acceptable.

Consider obedience and conformity from the patient's perspective. It could be suggested that there is a power imbalance between professionals with knowledge and resources, and that sometimes this imbalance brings out the need to conform, not to 'rock the boat'.

Why might sociology and psychology be relevant to your practice?

Taking an example from recent healthcare practice, we can see how lessons learned from sociology and psychology can inform our responses to difficult situations.

Case study: Mid Staffordshire NHS Foundation Trust Inquiry, March 2010

In 2010, Emily Cook (a health correspondent for a daily paper) reported that up to 1,200 patients may have died as a result of 'shocking' treatment at Stafford Hospital. This story was based on a report by the Healthcare Commission which stated that Mid Staffordshire NHS Foundation Trust had an appalling and chaotic system of patient care.

The Healthcare Commission (now the Care Quality Commission) had a role in examining the quality of care delivered by NHS organisations. The Commission's report argued that between 400 and 1,200 more people died than would have been expected during 2005 to 2008.

According to Cook, families described 'third world' conditions in the hospital, with some patients resorting to drinking water from flower vases because they were so thirsty. There were many examples of poor care and neglect. In one ward, 55 per cent of patients had pressure sores when only 10 per cent had sores on arrival.

The health minister at the time was concerned enough to order an inquiry. In a 452-page report, Robert Francis QC stated: It was striking how many [patients'] accounts related to basic nursing care as opposed to clinical errors leading to injury or death. *Many patients had their basic needs ignored (see the box below). The conclusion was that patients were* routinely neglected *in the context of cost cutting, targets and processes that lost sight of the basic need to provide safe care.*

Examples of patient neglect as found in the Mid Staffs NHS Foundation Trust Inquiry (Francis, 2010)

- Calls for help to use the bathroom were ignored.
- Patients were left lying in soiled sheets.

- Patients were left sat on commodes for hours.
- Patients were left unwashed – at times for up to a month.
- Food and drink were left out of reach.
- Family members had to feed patients.
- There was a failure to make basic observations.
- Pain relief was given late.
- Patients were discharged inappropriately.
- There were poor standards of hygiene.
- Families removed dressings and had to clean toilets.

The reasons outlined in the report for these deficiencies in care were as follows:

- *A chronic shortage of staff, particularly nursing staff, was largely responsible for the substandard care.*
- *Morale at the Trust was low.*
- *Many staff did their best in difficult circumstances; others showed a disturbing lack of compassion towards their patients.*
- *Staff who spoke out felt ignored and there is strong evidence that many were deterred from doing so through fear of bullying.*

The Trust's board was found to be:

disconnected from what was actually happening in the hospital and chose to rely on apparently favourable performance reports by outside bodies such as the Healthcare Commission, rather than effective internal assessment and feedback from staff and patients.

The Trust failed to listen to patients' concerns, *the Board did not* review the substance of complaints and incident reports were not given the necessary attention.

Quotes are from www.midstaffsinquiry.com

Implications of the Mid Staffs Inquiry report for nurses

The terms *compassion, safety, dignity* and *human rights* are central to the NMC standards, and are as much about the values of nursing as they are about the skills required for practice. While the Mid Staffordshire case may be an extreme example of the breakdown of care, it is important not to dismiss it as something that you, as a registered nurse, would never take part in. Given a particular set of circumstances, this sort of situation could occur anywhere.

It is all too easy to assume that nursing is purely about physical care, and that the problem at Mid Staffordshire was solely about this. However, there are more complex factors beyond physical care that result in whether care is good or poor. Many of these reasons stem from sociological and psychological contexts, and a knowledge of sociology and psychology can help us to understand what was going on in this case and perhaps to avoid similar incidents.

Activity 1.3   *Research and evidence-based practice*

Go the website **http://www.midstaffspublicinquiry.com/report** and read the executive summary from page 7.

Explore the evidence used to come to the conclusions about care.

Examine the NMC code of ethics: **http://www.nmc-uk.org/Publications/Standards/ The-code/Introduction**

Identify at least two NMC ethical standards that were breached at Mid Staffordshire.

There are some possible answers to this activity at the end of the chapter.

Even a brief look at this report demonstrates how far from standards some clinical practice was. To begin to understand how this happens, we need to understand ideas around culture and socialisation, social forces and how individuals react to them. Concepts such as managerialism, rationality and risk management might help us to understand how things go astray (Hillman et al., 2013; Goodman, 2014). We need to understand ideas around group conformity and obedience and how our value systems get distorted by the social setting.

It will be clear from the following that there is often an artificial divide between the two disciplines. Social and psychological 'forces' operate on both the patient and the nurse, and interact with each other to help to create a social and inner world of the mind. It is important to understand that this works both ways, i.e. the ways in which we go about thinking also create our social 'forces'.

Two key concepts in sociology – socialisation and culture – are relevant to what happened at Mid Staffordshire, and to considering the implications for your own nursing practice.

What is socialisation?

Staff at the Mid Staffordshire NHS Foundation Trust may have been socialised into a particular culture that was detrimental to good care. But what is meant by 'socialisation'? One possible definition is as follows:

> *We may understand the idea that we are born into a society that has certain rules of behaviour and we, as human beings, learn these rules through a process of socialisation. Socialisation simply means the various ways we learn how to be a human being and are taught the basic rules of society we live in.*
> (Goodman and Clemow, 2008, p. 78)

Socialisation is the process by which we learn the customs, norms, values, attitudes, beliefs, mores and behaviours of our society – in other words, how we acquire our culture. However, socialisation provides only a partial explanation for the acquisition of culture. People are not blank slates to be written on by our society. We are not robotic social actors blindly learning culture. Scientific research provides strong evidence that people are shaped by both social influences and their hard-wired biological make-up (Dusheck, 2002; Westen, 2002; Ridley, 2003; Carlson et al., 2005). Our genes alone do not determine our behaviour; they interact with the social environment. Society shapes us through socialisation, and we then become agents for socialising others.

The following activity asks you to consider your own socialisation.

Activity 1.4   *Reflection*

Think back to your first day at secondary school. How did you know how to behave with other pupils and with the teachers? How did you learn the formal (and informal) rules for being a pupil in class (i.e. how were you socialised as a pupil)?

Now identify just one aspect of your health and how it has been shaped by your socialisation. Consider, for example, alcohol consumption and the possibility that you (or someone who does drink) might develop problems relating to alcohol or being overweight.

There is an outline answer to this activity at the end of the chapter.

Socialisation shapes our behaviour in quite fundamental ways, to the extent that we begin to feel that we could not behave in any other way. Take a common student pastime: drinking. The use of alcohol in UK society is seen very differently from that in some other European societies. People living in France or Spain may well be socialised into very different views and habits on drinking wine. In the UK many 'feel' that going to the pub is very normal and to be expected, whereas their counterparts from a very devout Islamic background may not feel the same way. However, growing up as part of a cultural minority group may mean that British Muslims feel themselves being socialised into two different cultures, resulting in tension that will need to be resolved.

A related idea is that of 'occupational socialisation' – learning the customs of an occupation. Many occupations and professions have their own ways of speaking, dressing and behaving. Although almost 30 years old, Melia's (1987) study of the occupational socialisation of student nurses still sheds light on how we become the nurses we are, and illustrates the tension felt by students as they juggle the demands of education and the service needs of the NHS.

What is culture?

The shared beliefs, norms, values, attitudes, mores and behaviours of a society make up its culture. This involves language use, the way we dress, the food we eat, what leisure we like, whether work is valued – even what sports we value. Into this mix are ideas about dominant and subordinate cultures, or subcultures, within wider culture. Culture is dynamic and subjective. It changes over time, sometimes rapidly. It is defined by those who are experiencing it and will mean different things to different people. Therefore and from an understanding of how we become socialised into a culture, as described above, we may see that culture affects how we behave, our attitudes and our values. At Mid Staffs the organisational culture was described as having elements of:

- bullying;
- target-driven priorities;
- disengagement from management;
- low staff morale;
- isolation;
- lack of candour;
- acceptance of poor behaviours;
- reliance on external assessment;
- denial.

So it can be hypothesised that, despite professional codes of conduct (NMC, 2008), some nursing staff and care staff were socialised, perhaps against their will, into accepting poor practice. Although many staff did raise concerns, the organisational culture was such that not enough was done to prevent poor-quality care. Thus, culture overrode humanistic caring socialisation or perhaps reinforced an already accepted dehumanised socialised practice.

Socialisation and culture can be viewed as strong social forces that shape how we go about our business in an organisation. We may think we are completely free agents, making free choices, but the experiences of nurses at Mid Staffs shows that the culture can very seriously affect behaviour – in this case, the reporting of and delivery of inadequate care. Traynor (2014) also suggests that nursing failures are a possible inevitable consequence of the bureaucratic 'system' of care itself. The characterisation of nursing as primarily *character-based moral work*, with its emphasis on recruiting those with compassion, acts to block wider understanding of care failures, rooting them instead within the failing individual. Sociology moves us on from blaming individuals as the sole reason for poor care. Instead, it asks us to investigate the social processes that affect individuals in an attempt to devise solutions that go beyond the individual and focus as well on the nature and culture of organisations in which people have to work. Hillman et al.'s (2013) study illustrates this in action.

To really understand our social world and our individual lives we could use the 'sociological imagination'.

C. Wright Mills and the sociological imagination

C. Wright Mills was an American sociologist who argued that it was not enough merely to describe society: what was needed was an understanding that how we live our individual lives is shaped by the historical period in which we find ourselves, and the society we were born into. In turn, society develops out of the mass of individual lives. The sociological imagination is a way of understanding the relationship between history and personal lives so that we can understand that our personal experiences and 'troubles' are often linked to wider social issues: *men* [sic] *do not usually define the troubles they endure in terms of historical change* (Wright Mills, 1959, p. 3).

For example, a middle-aged man has a heart attack, a young woman develops an eating disorder, a teenager spends a night in accident and emergency with alcohol poisoning after a night out with his friends. None of these may consider their 'illness' to be linked to wider social issues. They are *seldom aware of the intricate connection between the patterns of their own lives and the course of world history* (Wright Mills, 1959, p. 4).

Lying in a hospital bed, with electrocardiogram electrodes stuck to his chest, the middle-aged man may curse his luck, or put his condition down to being overweight, his smoking habit and lack of exercise. The young woman feels that the only thing she controls in her life is her eating, becoming fixated on her dieting. The teen has not put much thought into binge drinking, and the industry that supports it and profits from it, other than not losing face with his friends. Wright Mills' arguments suggest that, without the sociological imagination they may not *possess the quality of mind essential to grasp the interplay of man and society, of biography and history . . . In addition, they . . . cannot cope with their personal troubles in such ways as to control the structural transformations that lie behind them* (Wright Mills, 1959, p. 4). But what does Wright Mills mean by a *structural transformation?*

Think of society as having 'structures', a class structure or a family structure (Parsons, 1955), which vary from society to society and which vary within the same society over time. These structures are created when individuals, groups, communities and populations act out their relationships with one another. Relationships between people both evolve as humans live their lives and also then act as structural patterns for others to follow. This process of 'evolution' and 'pattern' then changes over time and between societies. As outlined in the introduction, individuals thus are both shaped by these structured patterns of living and in living their lives they in turn shape the patterns (structures). In this manner our lives are structured, but not determined. See Figure 1.1.

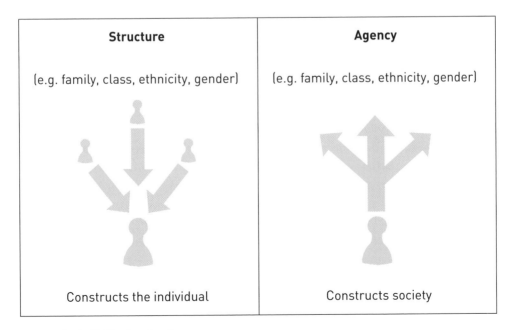

Figure 1.1: The individual and society

Activity 1.5   *Research and evidence-based practice*

Visit the Office for National Statistics (ONS) website and explore the different household types that currently exist in the UK: **http://www.ons.gov.uk/ons/dcp171778_393133.pdf**

To discover what the family structure in the UK looks like, start with asking: what is the most common family type in 2014? Google this question to find the ONS data.

There is an outline answer to this activity at the end of the chapter.

The ONS figures demonstrate that not everyone in the UK lives in the traditional nuclear family and thus question this as an ideal type. Social and geographical mobility, changing work opportunities and patterns, lifespan changes and attitudes to marriage and divorce have had their impacts on the type of family we can and wish to live in. This illustrates the changing structures of society.

To return to our earlier examples of the middle-aged man, the young woman and the teenager, what are those structures that lie beneath their personal troubles? To help answer that question, Wright Mills argues that what is needed *is a quality of mind that will help them to use information and to develop reason in order to achieve lucid summations of what is going on in the world and of what may be happening within themselves . . . this quality . . . [is] the sociological imagination* (Wright Mills, 1959, p. 5). The case study below illustrates this point.

Case study: The middle-aged man with a heart attack

A heart attack results from a variety of sources. Some may be genetic; others are patterns of living that are subject to social structures. The middle-aged man just happened to have been born in the 1950s into a working-class background (social class is a form of social structure). His father worked as a miner and he in turn followed in his father's footsteps. Living in a working-class town during the 1950s to the 1970s means engaging in certain eating habits, wearing certain clothes, taking holidays in certain places (only in the UK) and following certain sporting teams. And, of course, smoking. In this time period, smoking is as natural an activity as breathing – even professional footballers smoked. The 'metrosexual' man does not yet exist, there are no 'men's health' magazines, cigarettes are cheap, there are no laws banning smoking in public places. The idea of working out in a gym does not feature, except in the working-class boxing clubs. Olive oil and the Mediterranean diet exist only in the Mediterranean. Eating (saturated fat) red meat is masculine. 'Jogging' has not entered into the English language; exercise is for athletes or only takes place when playing Sunday football for the local pub team. Car use is becoming more common and cycling is in decline.

The social structure of this man's early years involves lifestyles that increase his chance of a heart attack, but he is not aware of all the connections. He thinks all his choices are his own, and is unaware that choice is limited and results from those chances handed out to him. His choices are also based on imperfect information and also upon the wishes of others who want him to make certain choices (e.g. the cigarette manufacturers). If the society in which he lives offers him the choice of A, B and C and he chooses A, he may think he has made a real choice. But what if there are choices F, G and H that he is not aware of through circumstance or that history has not yet provided?

In 1950, one could choose to smoke anywhere and the lack of a strong public health campaign and research evidence did not point to the deadly nature of the practice. The personal trouble of lung cancer or a heart attack following a lifetime of smoking has to be seen in the context of that history. Fast forward to 2015 and a new historical period. The public issue of millions dying of lung cancer has effected change in society and now impacts differently upon the individual as social structures have been transformed since the 1950s.

The sociological imagination enables its possessor to understand the larger historical scene in terms of its meaning for the inner life (Wright Mills, 1959, p. 5). Thus, the middle-aged heart attack victim who has this 'quality of mind' would understand his present trouble as linked to the context of 1950s Britain where working-class life took smoking for granted. He knows that all his friends smoked and that the likelihood of him smoking was high, given the social context and the time in which he lived. This is what Wright Mills was referring to when he argued that *[t]he first fruit of this imagination . . . is the idea that the individual can understand his own experience and gauge his own fate only by locating himself within his period, that he can know his own chances in life only by becoming aware of all those individuals in his circumstances* (Wright Mills, 1959, p. 5), and when he argued that *[t]he sociological imagination enables us to grasp history and biography and the relations between the two in society. That is its task and its promise* (Wright Mills, 1959, p. 6). The implications for nursing include the realisation that certain diseases arise as a consequence of how we live our lives, which in turn are often shaped by circumstances beyond our understanding or control. Therefore, blaming the victim for the development of a disease is not helpful. This realisation should also help us to understand why the public health role of nursing involves understanding social change as much as helping individuals to change their behaviour.

Wright Mills makes a distinction between personal troubles and public issues: the personal troubles of milieu and the public issues of social structure (Wright Mills, 1959, p. 8). We will now look at each in more detail.

Troubles

These occur within the individual's immediate experience and relationships. They relate to the individual self and to those areas of social life of which the individual is immediately, directly and personally aware. The description of what the trouble is and what the solutions are comes from the individual and within the scope of the individual's 'social milieu'. Troubles are a private matter; they are values that a person feels are threatened. The nurse who experiences stress at being 'short-staffed' and is unable or unwilling to see that a patient is dehydrating and lies in soiled sheets has a personal trouble.

Issues

These are matters that go beyond the local environment of individuals and their inner life. They result as an 'organisation' of many such situations into the structure and institutions of society. The countless individual social milieus overlap and create society at points in history. Issues are a public matter; issues threaten values held by the public. When this happens there may be public debate about what that value is and what really threatens it.

All over the UK, groups of teenagers are getting drunk on the streets and in other public spaces. There is an 'organisation' of all these incidents into an issue for the general public. The newspapers report on teenage drinking and the threat this poses, and discuss the various reasons for it. Public order is felt to be threatened by some; others debate that social cohesion and a loss of sense of community are at root; others discuss the role of the power of advertising, the cultural meaning of masculinity, the availability of cheap alcohol and the alcopops industry.

Wright Mills argues:

> Man's chief danger today lies in the unruly forces of contemporary society itself, with its alienating methods of production, its enveloping techniques of political domination, its international anarchy. (Wright Mills, 1959, p. 13)

These thoughts are echoed by Capra (1982), Hamilton (2003, 2010), Hopkins (2008), Jackson (2009), Worldwatch Institute (2010) and countless others. According to Wright Mills, *it is the task of the social scientist [and the liberal educationalist] to apply the sociological imagination to an analysis of the forces of social structure and to an analysis of how individuals' lives come together to construct a society that so threatens our existence.* To go back to our three examples, what is it about society that 'forced' working-class males to smoke and eat fatty foods? What is it about individuals' sense of who they are in that they choose to live an unhealthy cardiac lifestyle? What social structure makes a young woman starve herself and what meaning does a young woman bring to being thin? Why do some teenagers binge drink and why do they value drunkenness?

Patient experiences became public issues at Mid Staffs and moved beyond the personal trouble of a few individual nurses. We may ponder what was it about the local social structure that allowed care to be undertaken as it was. The report indicates that a particular management approach, as an aspect of social structure, underpinned some of the poor practices. Any nurse with a sociological imagination would be able to link their personal experiences of poor care with an analysis of the social context in which they work. This may be a necessary condition for change, but it may not be sufficient. The analysis may throw up issues of unequal power relationships that work against whistleblowing.

Sociology and public health

Health and illness can be thought of as arising from social structure as well as, if not more than, biology (Morrall, 2009). The knowledge that poor cardiac health results not just from the individual's choice of smoking and poor diet, but also from the social environment, indicates that nursing should, and does, have a public health role. Health education is not just an individually focused issue, based on a biomedical understanding. Health itself has social origins. For example, the concept of an 'obesogenic environment' suggests that we get fat because of the social environment we live in. It is not just about individual weakness and poor choice of lifestyle. The easy availability of cheap, high-sugar, high-calorie foods in our immediate surroundings, coupled with poor public transport in some areas and the growth of car use (Roberts and Edwards, 2010), has resulted in an increase in obesity.

Therefore, strategies that will assist people to move towards health must take into account the social context in which they live. Society has to change as much as the individual. Individualised models for change that ignore this will have less chance of success. The nurse must become, as the social scientist and the liberal educator, an agent for social change.

Nurses work with individuals and should understand that illness, although at first may seem self-inflicted out of free will, may result from the social milieu of the individual. Victim blaming of the unpopular patient, the self-harmer, the drug addict, the alcoholic is not only poor practice but is theoretically myopic; that is to say, it does not understand the social *causes of the causes* (Marmot, 2010) of illness.

Students in Mid Staffs may have worked in a social context of bullying and isolation and where poor practice became acceptable. They would have experienced these as personal troubles. The public issue is the organisational culture that arose that enabled this to take place. The Mid Staffs experience demonstrates that the standards of care demanded by the NMC were not upheld, but the social context suggests reasons why not. Just as it is not always right to blame a man for his heart attack, it may not be appropriate to blame students and staff as being solely responsible for poor practice.

This is a sociological discussion: what might psychology give us?

Social learning theory and moral disengagement

Behavioural theorists proposed that all behaviour is learned through a system of rewards or punishments. Albert Bandura and Richard Walters (1963) challenged this approach and set up an experiment to demonstrate that humans also learn by observing others (social learning theory). In his Bobo doll experiment, he tested the hypothesis that children who had watched aggressive behaviours would imitate their models when frustrated. His results are unsurprising and show that children who observed aggression will copy these behaviours when frustrated.

Bandura developed his theories concerning human aggression and proposed a theory of moral disengagement to explain how we convince ourselves that ethical standards do not apply to us. Like Zimbardo (2004), he considers a particular context is necessary to separate moral reactions from inhumane conduct. For him, the process of moral disengagement has four stages:

1. reconstructing conduct (the need to make 'bad' conduct 'good');
2. displacing responsibility;
3. disregarding injurious consequences;
4. dehumanising or blaming the victim.

These themes can help us explain what might have happened at Mid Staffs, as indicated in Table 1.1.

Reconstructing conduct	'We're short of staff and doing our best' So bad conduct becomes 'our best' because of poor staffing
Displacing responsibility	'Management don't care, it's their responsibility'
Disregarding injurious consequences	'There is not much I can do about this'
Dehumanising or blaming the victim	'It's his own fault he fell; I told him not to get out of bed' 'They're all senile and don't know what's happening anyway'

Table 1.1: Bandura's theory of moral disengagement at work in a nursing context

In the cold light of day, 'moral disengagement' would seem to be reprehensible, but that is the point. People learning from those they work with in very difficult situations can reconstruct acceptable behaviour by going through these stages and rationalising to themselves why care is as it is.

Humanistic psychology and the needs of the patient

The previous sections have examined psychological factors that impact on the way the care deliverer, i.e. the nurse, delivers care, but what about the patient's psychological state? Clearly, some of the nurses at the Mid Staffs hospital failed to recognise their patients as individuals with unique histories, feelings and worth. They could not see the psychological needs of their patients. This section will now consider how and why understanding the psychological needs of the patient is so important.

Much of the work in the psychological aspects of nursing care comes from the studies of Abraham Maslow (1954) and Carl Rogers (1961). They belonged to a group of humanistic psychologists who focused on the whole person, and the uniqueness of each individual. The theories of Rogers and Maslow have provided the foundation for the counselling and the human growth movement and are much referred to in nursing. At the heart of their studies was an emphasis on the importance of human emotion, known as 'affect', in driving thought and behaviour. Maslow believed that we are driven to achieve our full potential, which he called self-actualisation. Individuals are recognised as having different potentials. They may be blocked from the goal of self-actualisation by physical or psychological problems. If Maslow's theory is related to nursing, the role of the nurse could be said to be in assisting individuals to overcome the problem and allow progression. For example, a patient may have breathing difficulties, which denies her the opportunity to go out and socialise. By helping the patient overcome these difficulties the nurse allows her to progress towards achieving other things in her life. For example, a poet cannot write poetry if she is struggling to breathe following an asthma attack. Some patients have problems with their self-esteem, so the nurse can help the patient to examine their body image or self-perception in order to progress.

Maslow argued that there is a hierarchy of needs (Figure 1.2). Before we can achieve self-actualisation we need to meet more basic needs such as those for food, safety and shelter. During periods of acute illness, people need help to meet their physiological and safety needs. When a patient is chronically ill your role, in addition to helping with physical needs, is to provide care to help patients meet their needs for love, belonging, esteem and towards self-actualisation. Because chronic illness cannot be cured, it will affect a patient's daily living activities, sense of self and progression on the road to self-actualisation.

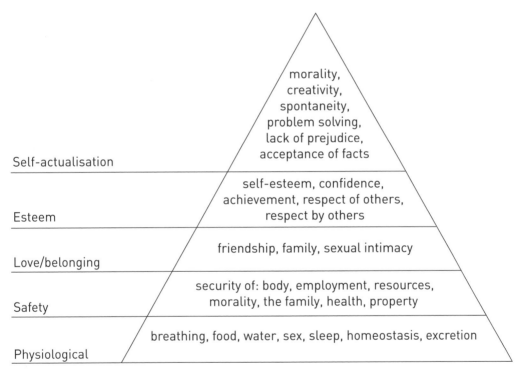

Figure 1.2: Maslow's hierarchy of needs

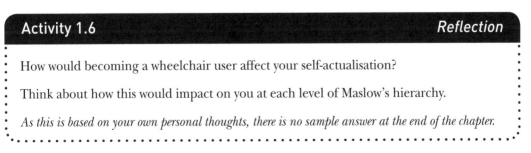

Activity 1.6   *Reflection*

How would becoming a wheelchair user affect your self-actualisation?

Think about how this would impact on you at each level of Maslow's hierarchy.

As this is based on your own personal thoughts, there is no sample answer at the end of the chapter.

Carl Rogers (1961) expanded on Maslow's theories. He believed that people became blocked in their development through faulty learning and self-doubt. He proposed that unconditional positive regard is essential to healthy development. He described this as acceptance and support of a person, regardless of what the person says or does. People who have not experienced it may come to see themselves in the negative ways that others have made them feel. Essentially, we learn to love ourselves by being loved. By providing unconditional positive regard, self-esteem is nurtured and the person learns confidence and trust.

Unconditional positive regard does not mean total acceptance of an individual. Rogers considers it is essential that we should say if a person's behaviour causes us to feel uncomfortable. It is the behaviour that is confronted, not the person. Regard is still given to the person through acknowledgement of the experiences that have produced the unpleasant behaviour, while the need for behavioural change is addressed.

Rogers advocates giving unconditional positive regard in the following ways:

- Genuineness: this requires honesty with the person through effective non-verbal and verbal communication.
- Empathy: the ability to feel what the client feels, which is different from sympathy and involves putting yourself in the patient's situation.
- Respect: the acceptance of the person as an individual.

By showing genuineness, empathy and respect to our patients we foster their self-esteem during periods of illness and adjustment. The NMC generic standards for competence in the domains of professional values, communication and interpersonal skills, and practice and decision making emphasise this aspect of care. The word 'compassion' is mentioned at least three times, as is the need to *promote optimum health*, to *promote health and well-being* and the need to assess and meet the *full range of essential physical and mental health needs*. The NMC is clear on this aspect, that nursing is about meeting *complex . . . needs in any setting*.

Findings from the inquiry at Mid Staffs clearly show that the care given did not even meet the lowest of Maslow's hierarchy (physical needs and safety). The problem is that clear codes of conduct exist, from the NMC for example, in addition to the NMC standards of competence. The question arises that, in spite of clear professional direction in written documents, staff were still unable to address the fundamentals of care. Sociological and psychological theory may help to understand the processes that were at work and understanding is the first step to changing practice. However, if individual behaviour is linked to how the group behaves, if a coercive culture exists that shapes how we think and act, then placing the burden of accountability upon the individual may be a little unfair. What was, of course, clear from the inquiry was that a breakdown of management set the tone for what followed. Clearly issues around leadership and management practices in the NHS require analysis (Hewison and Griffiths, 2004; Edmonstone, 2009; Hillman et al., 2013; Hutchinson and Jackson, 2013) to take us beyond blaming individuals.

The holistic therapeutic relationship

Sociology and psychology, as stated earlier, are seen as two distinct social sciences. However, it is the case that the areas of interest and study overlap. What is important, and the holistic therapeutic relationship illustrates this, is that care is composed of physical, psychological and social aspects (Lawler, 1991; Morrison and Burnard, 1997; Montgomery and Dossey, 2008).

We have briefly addressed the psychological needs of our patient above. However, the provision of holistic care requires us to address the patient's physical and social needs as well. Montgomery and Dossey (2008) advocate meeting patients' needs holistically through engagement in a therapeutic relationship.

Physical aspects of the therapeutic relationship

Few relationships outside the parental and intimate lead to such close physical contact as the therapeutic relationship between nurse and patient. These too involve sociological and psychological ideas such as 'taboo'. Lawler (1991) describes the embarrassment some nurses experience when first performing a blanket bath. In this situation we touch parts of the body that are usually private and only seen or touched by intimate relatives. Lawler considers that dealing with such encounters in a therapeutic way is part of the art and science of nursing. Nurses need to be able to observe and examine their patients without causing distress, while maintaining the patient's dignity. The therapeutic use of touch needs to be appropriate and varies with culture. Jourard (1966) found that certain areas of the body were taboo, but as nurses we deal not only with these taboo areas of the body but with body waste as well. Consider the rules around touch in the next activity.

Activity 1.7 — *Reflection*

If your tutor patted you on the head, how would you feel?

Would you feel patronised? Is such a gesture appropriate?

Consider the social rules that govern undertaking a rectal examination.

Consider the social rules that govern touching children.

Consider the social rules around restraining someone who exhibits challenging behaviour.

There is an outline answer to this activity at the end of the chapter.

Social aspects of the therapeutic relationship

A person's role can have a negative effect on cognition, affect (feelings) and behaviour (Zimbardo, 2004). However, role can also have a positive effect on a person's perception of him- or herself or others. In our culture, nurses have been generally perceived in a positive way. Within media depictions the nursing role has become associated with certain stereotypes (Ferns and Chojnacka, 2005). Stereotypes are over-generalisations about a group, which sometimes contain a grain of truth. Thus, 'all nurses are female' has an element of accuracy but ignores the fact that approximately 10 per cent of nurses are male. Stereotypes usually contain the words 'all' and 'are'. They can be positive or negative, but are more frequently associated with negative perceptions. In order to explore this further, undertake the following activity on nursing stereotypes.

Activity 1.8   *Team working*

Nurses have physical contact with their patients. Other workers have physical contact as part of their work. This may lead to a particular image of nursing (a stereotype) (Ferns and Chojnacka, 2005).

With two or three of your colleagues, list the stereotypical images of nurses you have encountered.

There is an outline answer to this activity at the end of the chapter.

Those of you old enough to remember the *Carry On* films may hold an image of the matronly Hattie Jacques. Part of 'Matron's' stereotype was as a spinsterly authority figure.

An advertising campaign in the UK ran with the slogan, 'Are you man enough to be a nurse?' This rests upon the idea that nursing is a female occupation, which in turn is based on the idea that it is 'natural' for women to care. So, to appeal to men, an appeal to intelligence, skill and courage is necessary as these are 'manly' traits. The stereotype of 'nurse as female and carer' has to be thus inverted to appeal to men. A new nursing role has to be created to ensure that men will be attracted to the profession. The new role creation, it is hoped, will create positive perceptions within men as nurses. The stereotype of nurse as female is thus unhelpful in recruiting men.

Patients can fall foul of stereotypes as well. Stereotyping denies individuality and confers some common characteristics to every individual who receives the label, such as 'diabetic' or 'elderly'. As nurses we need to see the patient as an individual person, not a diagnosis or one of a group.

Fiske and Taylor (1991) describe how over-generalisations or stereotyping can help us deal with the massive amount of information we are bombarded with in any social situation. Our cognitive systems can only process a limited amount of data at one time, so we focus on social cues such as gender, age, ability and ethnicity, to prevent information overload. This phenomenon, referred to as the 'cognitive miser', facilitates the quick processing of information. The downside is loss of individual data (Fiske and Taylor, 1991).

Stereotypes influence both perceptions and recall of others, even when we have not met them. Kelly (1955) found that when subjects were shown photographs of good-looking people they were more likely to describe them as intelligent or happy. This effect has become known as the 'halo effect' and is used to account for one trait dominating the perception of the whole person. Sadly, Kelly (1955) also found the converse to be true. Those described as ugly or disfigured were more likely to be judged as unintelligent.

Allport (1954) described prejudice as *an extreme and usually negative attitude made up from three components which are cognitive, affective and behavioural.* The cognitive aspect of prejudice is a belief based on false or incomplete facts, a stereotype. The affective or emotional component is strongly positive or negative, and provides the motivation that drives the behaviour. Allport describes five stages of prejudicial behaviour that have proved useful in examining and explaining the psychological factors that led, in extreme cases, to genocides like those in Rwanda and Bosnia. The five stages of prejudicial behaviour are as follows.

1. Antilocution: This means a majority group freely make jokes about a minority group. Speech is in terms of negative stereotypes and negative images. It is commonly seen as harmless by the majority. Antilocution itself may not be harmful, but it sets the stage for more severe outlets for prejudice. So, reflect on the use of words to describe older people. To what degree do care staff engage in antilocution, even in passing?
2. Avoidance: People in a minority group are actively avoided by members of the majority group. No direct harm may be intended, but harm is done through isolation (e.g. social exclusion). To what degree do we, as a society, isolate and avoid the older person?
3. Discrimination: The minority group is discriminated against by denying them opportunities and services, so putting prejudice into action. Behaviours have the specific goal of harming the minority group by preventing them from achieving goals, getting education or jobs. Sometimes, the majority group is actively trying to harm the minority, e.g. in apartheid. Do we currently deny those with learning disabilities, severe mental health issues, or the frail older person, opportunities and services? Does society, and individuals, engage in discriminatory practices?
4. Physical attack: The majority group vandalise, burn or destroy minority group property and carry out violent attacks on individuals or groups. Sadly, this has been documented in places such as Winterbourne View (see Chapter 2, Activity 2.3). However, this is not the action of the majority group.
5. Extermination: The majority group seeks extermination or removal of the minority group, such as ethnic cleansing in Bosnia. Thankfully, in the care context we do not go this far. However, can we think of 'extermination' existing not as a physical process, but as a mental or social one? To what degree have we removed certain groups of people from our normal social experiences and hence 'exterminated' them from our consciousness?

Allport's descriptions of prejudice may not have been at work at Mid Staffs, but considering the conditions there, it is at least possible that, within a management culture that put pressure on staff, the other normal psychological and social processes came together to create a culture of care that fell dangerously short of therapeutic.

Chapter summary

- Health and illness both derive from societal structures and psychological factors (as well as biology).
- The experience of health and illness has to be understood in the context of history, culture and social 'forces'.
- People have complex social and psychological needs.
- The meanings that people attach to health and illness are not only built by social structure but go towards creating social structures.
- Professionals need to acknowledge the complexity of health and illness and adopt a more open, non-judgemental viewpoint.
- Models for change have to go beyond individualised biomedical understandings of health and illness.
- Obedience and conformity can be shaped by the group.
- Individual values and judgements are not always derived from free will.
- People use short cuts such as stereotypes to understand others.

Activities: brief outline answers

Activity 1.2 Research and evidence-based practice

Students were asked to play the role of 'teacher'.

The 'treatments' applied were electric shocks at varying levels.

Sixty-five per cent of participants continued to apply the treatment despite the reactions they witnessed.

A possible flaw in the experiment is that the design does not take into account the fact that the actors knew the situation was not real. They may have been giving off unconscious non-verbal cues that the participants read as non-verbal clues.

Activity 1.3 Research and evidence-based practice

Two ethical standards which may have been breached are:

1. You must treat people as individuals and respect their dignity.

2. You must treat people kindly and considerately.

Activity 1.4 Reflection

As the first question is based on your own personal thoughts, there is no sample answer.

Social factors implicated in binge drinking include ease of access to alcohol, price, peer pressure, acceptance by mainstream culture, advertising and marketing, (student) rites of passage. Whether this leads to alcoholism may depend on various other factors, including genetic and other psychosocial factors.

Activity 1.5 Research and evidence-based practice

The married or civil partner couple without dependent children is the most common family type – 7.7 million.

Activity 1.7 Reflection

Patting someone on the head can be interpreted as a paternalistic ('father-like') action, based on a sense of traditional hierarchy. The father is 'superior' to, and is entitled to do this to, his young children. In Western culture patting a child on the head is seen as an affectionate gesture; when it is done to another adult it is perceived as patronising.

In each of the given examples about 'social rules' in sensitive situations, there are clear 'rules of engagement'. For example, while performing a rectal examination it would not be appropriate to have a colleague with you who was not needed for the activity and who engaged in discussions of a social nature.

Given the legislative framework and social issues around paedophilia, male nurses should not touch children without a chaperone.

Restraining people has strict guidance about whether it is appropriate and the level of force required. Certain techniques are prohibited but have been used in abusive practice in care homes.

Activity 1.8 Team working

Ferns and Chojnacka (2005) list the following stereotypes of nurses: angels and swingers, matrons and sinners. You may be able to think of some other terms, like battleaxe, doctor's handmaiden, bosomy matron.

Further reading

Denny, E and Earle, S (2010) *Sociology for Nurses.* London: Polity Press.
This book is useful for an indepth discussion on why sociology is relevant for nursing.

Gross, R and Kinnison, N (2013) *Psychology for Nurses and Health Professionals.* Boca Raton: CRC Press.
This book gives a good grounding in the relevant psychological theory.

Useful websites

www.nmc-uk.org

For the Nursing and Midwifery Council's code of ethics.

www.midstaffsinquiry.com

The report into Mid Staffordshire NHS Trust. Essential reading as background to this chapter.

www.soc.uu.se/research/research-projects/gerotranscendence

Lars Tornstam summarising his theory of gerotranscendence.

Chapter 2
Professional values

NMC Standards for Pre-registration Nursing Education

This chapter will address the following competencies:

Domain 1: Professional values

1. All nurses must practise with confidence according to *The Code: Standards of Conduct, Performance and Ethics for Nurses and Midwives* (NMC, 2008), and within other recognised ethical and legal frameworks. They must be able to recognise and address ethical challenges relating to people's choices and decision-making about their care, and act within the law to help them and their families and carers find acceptable solutions.

7. All nurses must be responsible and accountable for keeping their knowledge and skills up to date through continuing professional development. They must aim to improve their performance and enhance the safety and quality of care through evaluation, supervision and appraisal.

8. All nurses must practise independently, recognising the limits of their competence and knowledge. They must reflect on these limits and seek advice from, or refer to, other professionals where necessary.

Domain 3: Nursing practice and decision making

1. All nurses must use up-to-date knowledge and evidence to assess, plan, deliver and evaluate care, communicate findings, influence change and promote health and best practice. They must make person-centred, evidence-based judgements and decisions, in partnership with others involved in the care process, to ensure high quality care. They must be able to recognise when the complexity of clinical decisions requires specialist knowledge and expertise, and consult or refer accordingly.

Domain 4: Leadership, management and team working

3. All nurses must be able to identify priorities and manage time and resources effectively to ensure the quality of care is maintained or enhanced.

Chapter aims

After reading this chapter, you will be able to:

- give some definitions of professionalism;
- understand how concepts of professionalism are influenced by the prevailing society and culture;

- describe the different ways that professionals and patients relate to each other;
- show an awareness of the ethics of professional relationships.

Introduction

In the previous chapter we argued that insights from psychology and sociology may help in developing critical understanding of clinical practice and the context in which it takes place. We discussed how society and the way that individuals think and act are interlinked. We also suggested that the failures at Mid Staffs are a result of a complex set of factors and although at one level individuals may be blamed for poor care standards, to stop there would not do the issues justice. This chapter takes a critical look at the notion of professional values. Values can be discussed and listed; however, what professionals actually *do* needs critical examination.

To do this we need to investigate what we mean by 'professional' in sociological terms, and consider how professions operate in society. We need to examine the professional–patient relationship and consider what is ethical professional practice. Finally, we have to revisit what 'care' may mean.

What is 'professionalism'?

Activity 2.1	*Team working*

Students in clinical practice are assessed on a range of criteria. Mentors and assessors may comment on 'professional' or 'unprofessional' behaviour. In a small group, using a flip chart, discuss what you think is meant by these terms. Are there any contradictions or disagreements about what is meant by them?

An outline answer to this activity is given at the end of the chapter.

Analyses of professions initially rested on two main approaches: what *traits* are exhibited by professions and what *functions* do they perform for society? Both of these approaches can be traced back to the work of Emile Durkheim (Morrall, 2001), who tried to explain the need to control individuality within society in order to prevent societal disintegration. The argument made here is that the professions fulfilled a social role by acting in society's interest over and above their own, and in doing so encouraged social cohesion. The work they do in this view is vital for social functioning. The traits approach explains or describes what characterised the 'higher' professions – law, medicine and the clergy (Carr-Saunders and Wilson, 1933):

- altruism – professionals are motivated by the need to work for the public good;
- a specialised body of knowledge, which may be science-based in the case of medicine;
- an exclusive body of knowledge that no other occupation has;
- a lengthy vocationally orientated period of training;
- the ability, and authority, to self-regulate;
- a monopoly over its sphere of practice.

If an occupation is said to have these 'traits' and performs the function of promoting social cohesion, then it follows that the occupation might be a 'profession'.

Iatrogenesis and counterproductivity

This trait approach has been criticised for being a *description* of what professionals are and do *in theory* rather than in actual practice, and for omitting how power operates in society along either class or gender dimensions. Eliot Friedson (1970) debunks the trait and functionalist approach to understanding professions. Medicine, in Friedson's analysis, was *blind to its own shortcomings* and acted more in self-interest than in the interests of society. To this critique can be added Ivan Illich's ideas of iatrogenesis and counterproductivity. Iatrogenesis means 'brought forth by the healer' (Greek: *iatros* = healer; *genesis* = brought forth by) and so an iatrogenic disease/injury is one caused by medics. Illich argued:

> the pain, dysfunction, disability and anguish resulting from technical medical intervention now rival the morbidity due to traffic and industrial accidents and even war related incidents and make the impact of medicine one of the most rapidly spreading epidemics of our time.
> (Illich, 1976, p. 24)

Illich's critique may be an over-exaggeration of the negative impact of medical practice, but it does introduce the idea that professions may not always act in the public's interest.

Concept summary: Counterproductivity

Counterproductivity occurs when the institutions of an advanced industrial society reach a certain threshold and cease to be useful; their activities begin to go against their stated aims. A modern case may be care of the older person. Many frail older people are now 'cared for' in larger and larger care homes. The transformations in society that have required families to be mobile in search of work now result in the isolation of many elderly people from mainstream society, while society itself is struggling to come to terms with the costs of social care (Dilnot, 2011). The care industry, as it is becoming, may soon become counterproductive in the sense that the aim of providing a home and social care occurs in a context that militates against providing those aims to acceptable standards (Fahey et al., 2003; Royal College of Nursing, 2010; Care Quality Commission, 2014).

Care home companies state that the care their residents receive is more than adequate and that the Care Quality Commission (CQC) provides a measure of protection and quality for all residents. These companies would be unlikely to accept accusations of counterproductivity. However, it is the social institution and the social devaluation of care (Hagell, 1989) of which they are a part that could become counterproductive. More recently, the care of older people in acute hospitals has been criticised as lacking dignity (Hillman et al., 2013), while 'professional' management addresses risk at the expense of care (Goodman, 2014).

While developing the theory of counterproductivity, Illich collected statistics to support his case, so what is the evidence for this phenomenon today? The rise of evidence-based medicine (Sackett et al., 1996), it could be argued, is in part, or primarily, a response to practices that had little in the way of evidence to support their efficacy, as well as a result of a growing awareness of the damage some practices inflicted. It is important to distinguish between illness and injury caused by negligence and incompetence, e.g. surgical swabs left *in situ* after surgical closure, and that caused by the very practice of medicine itself when undertaken by its own rules and procedures. In addition, a distinction could be made between harm to individuals and harm to society. Harm to society may result in focusing on medical answers to social problems which deflect attention away from social answers. This latter point will be discussed in more detail later when we consider the inequalities in health issues (Marmot, 2010) and the social determinants of health approach (World Health Organization, 2008). An indication of the scale and types of harm caused to patients can be seen on the National Patient Safety Agency website: **www.npsa. nhs.uk**. Consider two areas that feature in the literature: medication errors and nutrition in hospital. You will be addressing both in detail during your course.

Iatrogenesis can be explored from a number of perspectives: clinical, social, cultural and technological. Clinical iatrogenesis involves physicians, surgeons and other healthcare professionals causing harm by negligence, incompetence and the application of techniques with questionable efficacy. Social iatrogenesis refers to the process by which *medical practice sponsors sickness by reinforcing a morbid society that encourages people to become consumers of curative, preventive, industrial and environmental medicine* (Illich, 1976, p. 49). It makes people hypochondriac and too willing to place themselves at the mercy of medical experts – a dependence on the medical profession that allegedly undermines individual capacities. The way society deals with death and dying are topics which may fall into this category and we will return to this later. Cultural iatrogenesis implies that societies weaken the will of their members by paralysing *healthy responses to suffering, impairment and death* (Illich, 1976, p. 49). Here, the whole culture becomes *overmedicalised*, with doctors assuming the role of priest, and political and social problems entering the medical domain.

Palmieri et al. (2007) outline technological iatrogenesis in addition to Illich's clinical, social and cultural iatrogenesis, in which modern healthcare has been characterised by a plethora of technologies, including information technology. These technologies, of course, enhance healthcare practice but, they argue, have introduced new ways of causing harm, which need to be addressed by risk management.

Professionalisation

Morrall (2001) suggests that a theme running through any examination of healthcare professions is the notion that medicine has been very successful in using professionalisation as a tactic for self-interest. We may suggest that nursing, however, in an attempt to become a profession, has not achieved quite the same protection and status, in part due to three things:

1. its subordinate relationship to medicine (Abbott and Wallace 1990);
2. its equivocal relationship to science;
3. the gendered nature of the profession in a culture that generally devalues female *emotional labour* (Smith, 1992).

Not only has nursing not emulated medicine's success in achieving the same status and privileges, but we may ask whether it should do so anyway. Emphasising 'caring' as a core value may be a way of differentiating nursing as well as creating its own professional identity. If we examine the three points above we may understand that nursing's professional path is complex in a world of changing cultural values and social transformation. Take the relationship to science. Nursing has not adopted scientific thinking wholesale into its knowledge and practice. It draws from science but also from other forms of knowledge, including some practices such as homeopathy. Society itself is characterised by various approaches to healthcare delivery, not all of which are science-based.

Concept summary: Professionalisation

It may be argued that trades, e.g. plumbing, and occupations, e.g. bank clerks, differ from professions as not being anything other than delivering competent skilled practice. However, if those working in trades and occupations attempt to establish themselves as having particular high-status values, e.g. integrity and trustworthiness, in society, then they engage in 'professionalisation'. This often involves establishing qualifications, often at degree level, to ensure a difference exists between the qualified professional and the skilled amateur. These qualifications are overseen by a professional body to regulate and set standards of professional conduct and then to establish group norms and acceptable modes of behaviour. The result is a divide between the knowledgeable professional and the client, who has to defer to that superior knowledge. 'Occupational closure' occurs when the profession then becomes closed to entry from outsiders, amateurs and the unqualified.

Why do occupations try to professionalise? It may be an attempt at gaining power, prestige, high income, high social status and privileges. Professions are thought to occupy a privileged elite status in society, demarcating themselves from common occupations. This then helps to ensure control by professionals over their own roles and members. It is thought that professional groups have access to powerful decision makers based on their superior education and knowledge.

Nursing: subordinate to medicine?

It is suggested that to be a true profession an occupational group must have autonomy over its own practice, that is to say, there is no other occupational group that supervises, guides, educates or directs its activities. Historically, nurses have worked a good deal under the supervision, guidance and direction of medics, and have even been educated by them. Therefore, to become a profession nursing must attempt to work autonomously as much as possible but in partnership with medics and other health professions. Abbott and Wallace suggested in 1990 that nurses were subordinate to medicine; today, we need to consider whether that interpretation has changed. Historically, medics diagnosed and prescribed treatments while nurses carried out tasks in relation to them, and this has been termed the handmaiden role.

In the latter half of the twentieth century, nursing has tried to carve out its own sphere of influence separate from medicine, emphasising its caring role over the curing role of medics. Nursing has taken control over supervision, direction and education. Ironically, in the attempt to identify its own sphere of practice, nursing has taken on many medical tasks partly directed by policy changes from the Department of Health.

Nurses and paramedics in certain clinical areas for example, minor injury units, now undertake:

- consultation interviews (taking a patient's history);
- performing clinical examination techniques (for example, inspection, palpation, percussion and auscultation of the chest);
- ordering, and in some cases, interpreting clinical investigations such as X-rays;
- deciding upon a range of possible diagnoses (differential diagnosis);
- implementing a treatment and management plan that may include prescribing medications.

To lay people it would only be the name badge, uniform or clinical setting that would indicate that it is a nurse and not a medic they are seeing. The question remains: in the development of some nursing roles, which are beginning to look more and more like medical practice, is nursing achieving the same status and privileges accorded to the medical profession? In any case, from a patient's perspective the status of nursing as a profession is not the issue; rather it is the primacy of caring (Benner, 1988). As long as they get the care they need, many patients are not bothered about the status of the profession.

Is nursing still subordinate to medicine? While it is true that nurses are now undertaking medical tasks and making independent decisions, sometimes without recourse to medics, it is still the case that legally the care of the patient is ultimately the medics' responsibility. Complex cases will still be referred to medics and policy decisions around, for example, healthcare reforms will still defer to medics as the primary profession.

A scientific underpinning to nursing knowledge?

It may be argued that important in becoming a true profession is the adherence to a scientific body of knowledge that legitimises medical practice for society. This sets medicine apart from 'quack' medicine and 'caring' practices. Nursing may have an uneasy relationship to science, both accepting it as a body of knowledge, but also wary of having nursing practice completely dominated by it. This is the second point regarding achieving status and privilege within society. Medicine historically has co-opted scientific understanding to legitimise its practice and continues to police the borders in an attempt to keep quack practice (pseudoscience) at bay. To get an understanding of this, visit Dr Ben Goldacre's site (**www.badscience.net**) or read his book *Bad Science* (Goldacre, 2008). This point will be revisited later in Chapter 5.

Concept summary: Pseudoscience

The word 'pseudo' is Greek for fake. Pseudoscience is knowledge, assertion, theory and hearsay masquerading as science and has the following characteristics:

- an indifference to facts – the literature spouts 'facts' that may not be so;
- the research it does is not systematic or rigorous and jumps to conclusions too easily;
- it starts with an appealing theory (hypothesis – e.g. water has memory) and then looks for things to support it rather than trying to disprove it;
- it does not use valid rules of evidence; instead, it appeals to eye witnesses, testimony, stories;
- it relies on subjective validation – 'it worked for me'.

For a full discussion, see **www.quackwatch.org** and type 'pseudoscience' in the search box.

In an attempt to be different from medics, and perhaps with a degree of suspicion about the total merit of scientific medicine when it comes to matters of health, some nurses have turned to complementary medical therapies to augment their own practices. This is also in line with the public's increasing tendency to use these alternatives as medicine and the opinion of experts becomes more challenged.

We may be entering an era in which the tenets of science and the status it affords its practitioners are increasingly being challenged by the public. Despite these challenges, however, scientific medicine is still the basis of prestige and status. The public still wants scientific and technological medicine. By embracing both science and non-science alternatives, nursing seeks status and privilege in both camps.

Activity 2.2   *Research and evidence-based practice*

To what degree are nurses engaging in practising complementary and alternative medicine (CAMs) and therapies? Are there specific clinical areas in which this happens?

> When you are next in clinical practice ask your colleagues what they think about the use of CAMs.
>
> Undertake a small literature search using the search terms 'nursing' and 'complementary therapy', 'alternative therapy', or use a term such as 'homeopathy' and 'nursing'. Does the size of the list you come up with (large or small) surprise you?
>
> *An outline answer to this activity is given at the end of the chapter.*

Care as emotional (women's) labour

The profession of nursing holds dear to a notion of 'care' as a core value of the profession. It is mentioned so often that referencing the fact is unnecessary. Emotional labour can be seen to be an aspect of what care may mean and could be seen as the antithesis – the opposite – of self-interested professionalisation. Thus, looking at it positively, care as emotional labour is something that nursing, perhaps arrogantly, uses to set itself apart from medicine. On the other hand, emotional labour is what is left when no other domain can be claimed as nursing's sole domain of practice. Or, it could be seen as just a manifestation of the devaluing of nursing by society because nursing is care work, care is women's work and society does not value women's work (Sullivan, 2002).

Smith and Gray (2001) argued:

> *Hochschild (1983) suggests that emotional labour involves the induction or suppression of feeling in order to sustain an outward appearance that produces in others a sense of being cared for in a convivial safe place. Emotional labour is typified by three characteristics: face-to-face or voice contact with the public; it requires the worker to produce an emotional state in another; it allows the employer through training and supervision to regulate a degree of control over the emotional activities of workers (Hochschild, 1983; Smith, 1992, p. 7). James (1993) describes emotional labour as skilled work requiring experience, affected by immediate conditions and external controls which connects public life with the private household and uncovers its paid and unpaid nature. Because of its association with women's work it is often rendered invisible and undervalued.*
> (Smith and Gray, 2001, p. 230)

Emotional labour describes much of what nurses are called to undertake and may be seen by the public in the absence of pay and high status as its own reward (see Theodosius, 2008, for research on emotional labour). Non-registered staff, i.e. healthcare assistants, are called to this work as well for even less pay and status than registered staff. In this context it may be suggested that many people are not able to give of themselves continually without experiencing stress and burn-out and for little public recognition or respect beyond the worn-out 'angels' epithet which, in any case, no longer applies, in the light of Mid Staffs and Winterbourne View, to name just two media-highlighted cases.

Activity 2.3   *Critical thinking*

Go to the Department of Health website and read the Review of Winterbourne View Hospital: **www.dh.gov.uk/health/2012/02/review-of-winterbourne-view-hospital**

At Winterbourne View (BBC, 2011a) residents were subjected to physical and emotional abuse. The situation occurred because of poor training, recruitment, management and supervision of staff, coupled with poor-quality inspection by the CQC, which subsequently was hit with a no-confidence vote by delegates at the National Care Homes Congress (Hill, 2011). The CQC argued that it considered the concerns raised by some staff were being dealt with at local level. In addition, and at about the same time, staff in care homes in Cornwall were urged to meet up with the CQC as they pronounced that many older people were suffering because of a lack of basic care and dignity (BBC, 2011b).

To what extent is this a result of care being so devalued that it is left to poorly trained, poorly supervised and poor in number staff? Why does care not have a higher status and thus higher preparation, supervision and pay in society? Why can nurses enter education with very little in the way of educational preparation compared to other professions – professions which in any case would not tolerate such (low) entry requirements (Shields et al., 2011)?

An outline answer to this activity is given at the end of the chapter.

A feminist critique of professionalisation

Wuest argues that *[t]he evolution of nursing knowledge and nursing as a practice discipline has been stunted by the quest for professionalism* (1993, p. 357).

The traits approach is based on male assumptions about what a profession is, and thus projects on to us what men think a profession should be. Thus, if nurses copy the strategies and 'ways of knowing', e.g. the use of objective empirical science, of other male-dominated professions, they merely reproduce male practices and male values, which women will always struggle to emulate (Wuest, 1993). A feminist outline of professional values would be based on the different ways of understanding the world and human relationships that it is argued women have. A difficulty, and a recognition of this, is that society is patriarchal – male-dominated – and success is only measured by male standards.

Carol Gilligan's (1982) work suggests that women construct a primary definition of themselves by their ability to care, and that they do so accepting the primacy of human relationships in their experience. However, men, including scientists, theorists and medics, have assumed that the care role is primarily female and have devalued this trait, seeing it as a weakness rather than as a strength. Gilligan argues that theories of psychology and economic development developed by men have this idea at their core. Further, it is suggested that the very traits that define what is good in women are seen and defined as deficient in moral development in the psychological literature.

Similarly, Hagell (1989) questioned the direction in which the nursing 'profession' was moving. The uncritical acceptance, defining nursing as a science and developing a scientific knowledge base, needed to be challenged. The argument here is that many of the basic assumptions about science, scientific method and scientific knowledge are partial understandings of what human relationships and caring actually are. Nursing, as a discipline, has a distinct knowledge base, which is not grounded in science and its methodology, but which stems from the lived experiences of nurses as women and as nurses involved in caring relationships with their clients.

This argument about the differences in male ways of thinking and values and female ways of thinking and values often sits behind and is implicit in other discussions about what the nursing profession should be and what its values are. A coming together of patterns on understanding nursing practice was outlined by Barbara Carper (1978).

Activity 2.4   *Research and evidence-based practice*

What evidence can you find to support the contention that medicine often acts in its own interests, and actually results in harm to many patients? Then consider to what degree this applies to nursing. Consider to what degree the actions by nurses at Mid Staffs were the result of burnout due to emotional labour.

Read the Francis report. Do you think there is any evidence in this to support that theory?

An outline answer to this activity is given at the end of the chapter.

A critique of the professional role for nursing

The espoused theory, i.e. what we say we will do, of nursing can be found in many places, but of course particularly within the pages of Nursing and Midwifery Council (NMC) *Standards for Pre-registration Nursing Education*. The 2010 standards emphasise a public health role and a focus not just on individuals but also on communities and population health. Implicit in the standards is the notion that this is about UK populations, as this is the jurisdiction of the NMC. The health needs of non-UK populations are not explicitly mentioned.

A critical view of the profession of nursing, following on from the works of Illich, Friedson and feminist theory, suggests that in reality nursing as a whole works using a mainly biomedical understanding of disease care. Nursing is a 'discipline of disease', focused on the individual at the expense of concerns with the health of communities and populations. The outcome of this is that nursing alongside medicine has abrogated its moral responsibility for health, which results in the misdiagnosing of the root causes of disease, often applying the wrong treatments to many illnesses within a *pharmaceuticalisation* (Williams et al., 2011) discourse as social and cultural iatrogenesis.

> ## Concept summary: Pharmaceuticalisation
>
> The pharmaceutical–industrial complex refers to the relationship between policy and finance engaged in between legislators, pharmaceutical companies and medical practitioners. These relationships may include political lobbying, to try to get beneficial legislation and oversight of the industry. It also includes marketing to medics and the application of drugs to problems as first-line treatments. A discourse arises when these practices become so accepted by the public that it seems just common sense to seek drug solutions to what are often social or life problems.
>
> *Pharmaceuticalisation* refers to the process, including:
>
> * the redefinition of health 'problems' so as to have a pharmaceutical solution (a pill for every 'ill');
> * the creation of new consumer markets;
> * drug innovations;
> * the mobilising of consumer and patient groups around drugs.

If we take the view that health is a global ethical issue, then it could be argued that professions have a moral responsibility for promoting health in all communities, including the health of the *bottom billion* (Collier, 2007). However, the charge is that many health professionals actually work within a system that provides care for those who are:

* suffering from the indulgences of consumer culture;
* 'cosmetically' challenged (as society defines what is beauty);
* self-centredly sad (rather than those with real mental health problems).

We all live in a global society – the interconnections are social, economic, cultural and ecological; individuals are interdependent on a finite planet (Goodman, 2011c). If this is accepted, then health is not an individual or local issue alone – it is a global social issue. We live in a messy world (Peccie, 1982; Morrall, 2009) in which inequalities in health are based on socioeconomic, ethnic and gender divisions. Because we know how to sort out this mess – we have enough understanding of the root causes of disease – we nurses have a moral obligation to do so through collective action. Questions remain: Are nurses too disillusioned and/or distracted to get involved? Is there a lack of professional and individual activism and radical intellectualism? Later chapters will address the social determinants of health approach (World Health Organization, 2008), which provides a theoretical and empirical background for action by nurses. The challenge will be to allow individual liberty to flourish while addressing the social causes of illness.

Activity 2.5   *Reflection*

Cecil Helman once reflected:

> *many children die young from infections, accidents, malnutrition, diarrhoeal diseases,*
> *many of them the diseases of poverty made worse by poor education . . . I think . . . of the*
> *hundreds of hours I've spent over the years [as a UK-based GP] on sniffles, colds, minor*
> *blemishes and invisible rashes, all those lengthy talks only about trivia.*
> (Helman, 2007, p. 181)

Consider this statement in the light of your experience of nursing practice.

As this activity is concerned with your own experiences and reflection, no outline answer is given.

The professional–patient relationship

The relationship between professionals and patients has been called paternalistic. However, it is argued that this is changing and that the patient should now be at the heart of the care system as a full partner in all care decisions. Goodman and Clemow (2010) outline some of the changes to health policies that underpin a patient-centred NHS, and you will need to access other sources that discuss the policy changes in detail. This includes patient and service user involvement policies. Go to the Royal College of Nursing's website and look up the theme Patient Focus: **http://www.rcn.org.uk/development/practice/clinical_governance/patient_focus**.

You will need to reflect on the care experiences and relationships that you will see around you as professionals go about their work and undertake a critique of decision-making processes that may appear to be paternalistic. This involves a certain ethical approach to care, which primarily focuses on the two ethical principles of autonomy and beneficence. 'Autonomy' entails having the freedom to make decisions for oneself, while 'beneficence' means 'to do good'.

Pater is the Latin word for father. A father wants the best for his children and will make decisions on their behalf because he thinks that the child cannot have the information or emotional maturity to make the right decisions. 'Paternalism' invokes the concept of care and authority (Robb, 2004). If professionals want 'to do good' (beneficence) and think they know what is best for the patient, then this could erode the patient's autonomy. The term 'doctor knows best' illustrates a paternalistic attitude and when health professionals make decisions on behalf of patients in what they consider to be, and actually may also be, their best clinical interests, they may act paternalistically.

According to Williamson et al. (2010), the 'doctor knows best' view is currently outdated and new approaches of working have been introduced within UK health policy (Goodman and

Clemow, 2010). Whether 'patient and service user involvement' policies have changed actual clinical practice requires some further investigation.

Upton et al. (2011) in a small study conclude that there is a misalignment between clinical practice and the 'rhetoric' regarding patient empowerment, questioning shared decision making, and thus implying paternalism in nursing consultations still exists. If this is the case, it is not surprising, due to long-held beliefs flowing from beneficence: the 'need to do good' outweighs the actual practice of sharing decisions and empowering patients. McKinnon (2014) however argues for the value of 'concordance' and moving away from paternalism even in clinical settings where patients' capacities for shared decision making may be compromised.

This wish to act in the best interest is to act with beneficence (to do good); when it overrides the patient's autonomy it becomes paternal. Nurses are urged to act ethically by the NMC and part of this practice is to recognise ethical practice by reference to some ethical theory, such as that outlined by Beauchamp and Childress (2009) or that of the *libertarian paternalism* outlined in *Nudge* (Thaler and Sunstein, 2008).

The sick role

Expectations of the patient and professional roles can be identified within the notion of the *sick role* (Parsons, 1951). The sick role outlines obligations and rights for patients to legitimise their status as sick. Parsons' perspective sees illness as deviance from the social norm. When people fall ill they perform the 'sick role' to legitimise that illness.

Society cannot function with illness unless it is legitimised. Successful performance of the sick role confers two rights:

1. the right to exemption from performing normal social roles;
2. the right to freedom from responsibility for their own illness.

However, there are also two obligations:

1. to want to get well speedily;
2. to consult expert medical opinion.

Doctors and nurses are involved in this role and have obligations to:

- apply a high degree of skill and knowledge to illness;
- act in the welfare of the patient, not their own self-interest;
- be 'objective' and emotionally detached and non-judgemental;
- be guided by rules of practice and code of conduct.

Unless the obligations are met, the right cannot be conferred and the result is illegitimate sickness. This model of the medic–patient relationship contains therefore elements of paternalism inherent within it.

Activity 2.6   *Reflection*

Identify an occasion when you were ill. Describe how you met the rights and obligations of the sick role. What implications does this have for you, your family and workplace? Identify groups of people who, because of their 'illness', cannot (will not?) fulfil their obligations.

As this activity is concerned with your own experiences and reflection, no outline answer is given.

Weaknesses of the 'sick role' as an idea

The 'sick role' does not address culture, gender, sexuality, race or class, chronic illness, mental illness or the experience of women and childbearing.

Parsons is uncritical of inequalities in the role of healthcare staff as gatekeepers and agents of social control. Patients are expected to be submissive and unquestioning of the medics' protective decision making to avoid harm and distress. In other words, the lay public relies on healthcare staff to legitimise their withdrawal from functioning in society. Withdrawing from 'normal' social roles may incur sanctions but this is avoided with 'sick notes'. However, only medical and nursing staff are seen to have this right to confer illness and withdrawing. In addition, this perspective does not discuss that functioning within society itself can make someone ill. This idea will be explored in more detail later.

A question arises as to whether certain groups within society are more likely to be treated paternalistically based on assumed group characteristics. Historically, within learning disability practice there was evidence of paternalism which considered the professional as powerful – paternalism has tragically, of course, turned into abuse in the recent case mentioned above – beneficence became maleficence: 'to do harm'. There was a belief that people with learning disabilities were 'eternal children' who lacked skills or understanding to make decisions regarding their own care until self-advocacy groups such as People First put them in charge of their own lives (Hannon and Clift, 2011).

Stewart et al. (2005) outline three approaches to decision making:

1. The paternalism model of care, whereby professionals hold the information and take responsibility for making decisions for their patient.
2. The shared decision-making model, which involves the professional and patient sharing information and involvement and responsibility for healthcare decisions.
3. The informed consent model, whereby it is the patients' responsibility to be fully informed on aspects of their healthcare and for any decision made.

In official pronouncements there is evidence of a shift away from a paternalism model towards a shared model of decision making. Robb (2004) suggested a few reasons for this:

- Social class differentials between medics and patients are less influential. The old sick role attitude of patients 'knowing their place' is no longer acceptable within healthcare practice, despite the existence of social inequalities in education, employment and income, which could potentially strip individuals and groups of their power *vis-à-vis* professional groups (Robb, 2004).
- It is also suggested that the information revolution and the birth of the internet have contributed to the shift of power whereby patients are now 'experts' in their own care.
- Media investigations, patient group pressure and internal competition have all contributed to the need for holistic patient-centred care, which respects the values and rights of individuals (McCormack and Corner, 2003).

Nevertheless, inquiries into the scandal surrounding the high child mortality rate at Paediatric Cardiac Services in Bristol suggest a paternalistic attitude leading to lack of informed consent, honest information, ineffective communication and poor counselling (Sheaff, 2005). Scandals such as this have knocked public confidence (Robb, 2004). More recent descriptions of care practices also demonstrate the power imbalance between people and professionals (Hillman et al., 2013). The document *Liberating the NHS: No Decision About Me Without Me – Government Response* (Department of Health, 2012a) clearly accepts that this is a goal rather than a description of actuality.

Professional 'care'

As already noted, 'care' is seen as central to healthcare practice, but there may be a difference between what is said and what actually happens. This is not just about lack of dignity and respect, or incompetence, but also what 'care' actually means to individuals. For some, the technical bio-medical aspects of care are foremost in their tacit theory of caring; for others, the principles of humanistic caring are to the fore. We can think about care delivery as crudely being based on four different ways of understanding health and illness:

1. the biomedical model – based on scientific medicine;
2. the biopsychosocial model – a holistic approach drawing upon social sciences as well as medicine;
3. the salutogenic model – a focus on health and what makes us healthy;
4. the complementary and alternative medicine model – the use of various treatments and therapies.

For an exposition of these approaches, go to **http://www.open.edu/openlearnworks/course/view.php?id=1319%3f**.

Perhaps the context affects how care is actually practised. Highly technical environments and emergency situations call for a certain skill set based on biomedical approaches, while long-term settings, clients in their own homes, clients in nursing care homes or palliative care settings will call for other skill sets in which care is practised. These may draw from the other three models of health delivery.

Professional nursing then may have an eclectic approach to healthcare delivery and however could still be practitioner-led.

What we have not focused on is that care is most often undertaken by family and friends in the community and is unpaid and undervalued. Sue Gerhardt, in *The Selfish Society* (2010a), addresses this theme of caring and argues that modern child-rearing practices result in acquisitiveness, emotional suppression and a lack of emotional development. Child-rearing practices then link with consumerism to produce a selfish society in which care is marginalised and under pressure from the need to earn a living. The pressure for women to go back to work too early results in the neglect of child care and development. This lack of emotional development leads many in society, including those at both the bottom and at the top, e.g. the finance sector, to have less empathy or connection with others. Therefore, capitalism has skewed values away from human connectivity, and an ethic of care based on a relational approach to each other. Child development, however, is a crucial aspect for a healthy society and is a key objective of an important report on health inequalities: *Fair Society, Healthy Lives* (Marmot, 2010). An express implication is that society should invest in the 0–3-year-olds to enable them to grow up in safety, love and emotive-relational development. Also, care should be formally recognised as a social function, as other social functions are, and that is by paying for it. This suggests that there is a cultural shift away from care and empathy, but more importantly, that child rearing results in a lessened ability to care.

Finally, Griffiths et al. (2012) investigated users' and carers' views on what they want to see in graduate nurses. The findings, although from a small qualitative piece of research, resonate with other expressed views on what caring may be (Finfgeld-Connett, 2008). In addition to technical competence, knowledge and the professional's willingness to seek information, a priority was *a caring professional attitude*, which of course gets us nowhere unless you unpick what that means. In the context of this study, this meant:

* empathy;
* communication skills;
* non-judgemental patient-centred care.

These attributes are often invisible to auditing procedures; it is not easy to measure them, nor to quantify or to develop 'targets' for them; nor is it easy for them to be defined as 'outcomes'. However, patients and nurses know what these things are. In an increasingly technical rational world (Goodman, 2011a), where the ends have to be measured and financially justified, invisible 'care', because it is invisible, is undervalued.

'Care' and the professional–patient relationship are ongoing issues, and possibly always will be, involving action by governments.

The 2014 Secretary of State for Health, Jeremy Hunt, and the Minister for Care and Support, Norman Lamb (The Stationery Office, 2013) wrote that the Care and Support Bill (2013) is based on a need to drive up the quality of care following the findings of the Francis inquiry. The law needs to refocus on: the needs of the person, not the service; improving carers' access to support; and introducing a new adult safeguarding framework. They argue that *patients are the first and foremost consideration of the system and everyone who works in it* to restore the NHS to its core values (The Stationery Office, 2013, p. 7). They clearly argue: *Today's care and support system often fails to live up to the expectations of those who rely on it . . . the system can often be confusing, disempowering and not flexible enough to fit around patients' lives* (p. 9). So, while not pointing directly at poor professional practices, the tone of the argument implies systemic failures which professional, clinical and managerial staff have not been able to address.

For nurses, a response since the Francis inquiry has been the development of the 6Cs approach, led by the Chief Nursing Officer. This is the Compassion in Practice initiative which highlights six enduring values and behaviours that underpin compassion in practice (Department of Health, 2012b). The 6Cs appear to be another clarification of what care is and follows on from previous work, such as the latest *Essence of Care* benchmarking exercises (Department of Health, 2010a) which themselves are refreshments of earlier work in 2001. All of this seems to indicate what to some might seem the 'obvious' and the fact that it needs spelling out in such terms might indicate something is lacking in the system.

The conclusion might be that professional caring operates in particular contexts that either hinders or helps what professionals can do. The Francis reports clearly demonstrated what certain contexts of target and financially driven managerial responses can do to both the practice of nursing and the experience of care ordinary people sometimes have to 'endure'.

Research summary: Defining care

Finfgeld-Connett (2008) looked at 49 research reports and six publications analysing the concept of care to try to define what caring is. The author concluded that care is a complex interplay of:

- expert nursing practice (involving assessment, knowledge and technical competence);
- interpersonal sensitivity (centring completely on the patient, non-judgementally and with openness and availability);
- intimate relationships (deep involvement with patients and families, sharing personal thoughts and feelings, but avoiding crossing the line into a personal relationship).

Chapter summary

- Nursing sees itself as a profession, but what this actually means is open to debate.
- Professional values are open to critique in that there may be elements of self-interest and they may be based on male assumptions.
- Professionals may have acted as if 'they know best', but policy now requires that the patient is at the centre of decision making.
- Care is a central value for professional nursing, but what that actually means may be open to interpretation and affected by the context in which it operates.

Activities: brief outline answers

Activity 2.1 Team working

As this is group work you will produce your own ideas, but they may include:

- turning up for work on time;
- wearing appropriate clothing;
- using appropriate language;
- being respectful to senior colleagues;
- not discussing personal matters with patients.

Some items on this list may be more about subordinate positioning than being a professional; a key concept is having autonomy to make decisions.

Activity 2.2 Research and evidence-based practice

You will find that many nurses have undergone training in one or more complementary therapies, and have attempted to import them into their clinical practice.

See: **Running, A and Turnbeaugh, E** (2011) Oncology pain and complementary therapy. *Clinical Journal of Oncology Nursing,* 15 (4): 374–379:

> *Half of all patients with cancer experience some level of pain, so pain management is an important topic for oncology nurses. Pharmacologic measures traditionally are the primary intervention for bone, visceral, neuro-pathic, and procedural pain; however, many patients are turning to an integrative approach of Western and complementary therapies for pain and symptom management. The authors explored the current evidence concern-ing the effectiveness of complementary therapies in relation to cancer pain and symptom control.*

Activity 2.3 Critical thinking

To answer these questions you will need to think critically about how and why society highly rewards and supports various occupations, for example that of 'Law'. Is it because of the gendered nature of caring, i.e. that it is seen as naturally women's work, and also as work that, therefore, needs little education to perform it? Certainly, feminist theorists would argue that is the case (see Hagell, 1989). You might want to think about the idea of 'professional closure' and control in the profession as discussed in the text. That is to say, some professions can very tightly control who gets in and the sorts of rewards they get.

Activity 2.4. Research and evidence-based practice

The answers to some of the questions in this activity will be based on your own findings and experience. However, the Francis report contains the following findings, which may be seen as evidence to support the theory that nursing actions at Mid Staffs were at least in part the result of staff burnout resulting from emotional labour:

> *attitudes of patients and staff – patients' attitudes were characterised by a reluctance to insist on receiving basic care or medication for fear of upsetting staff. Although some members of staff were singled out for praise by patients, concerns were expressed about the lack of compassion and uncaring attitude exhibited by others towards vulnerable patients and the marked indifference they showed to visitors.*

> *low staff morale – the constant strain of financial difficulties, staff cuts and difficulties in delivering an acceptable standard of care took its toll on morale and was reflected by absence and sickness rates in particular areas.*
> (Francis, 2010, p. 15)

Further reading

Friedson, E (2006) *Professional Dominance: The Social Structure of Medical Care.* Edison, NJ: Aldine Transaction.

Friedson continues to analyse the professional–lay person relationship to suggest power imbalances based on certain ideological assumptions.

Theodosius, C (2008) *Emotional Labour in Health Care.* Abingdon: Taylor & Francis.

This book looks at recent research on emotional labour.

Williamson, G, Jenkinson, T and Proctor-Childs, T (2008) *Contexts of Contemporary Nursing.* London: SAGE.

A wide variety of factors impact on the scope of nursing practice, including government policies, organisational structures, the media, education, future healthcare directions and service users themselves. This book provides a clear and practical introduction to these contexts for the new nursing student.

Useful websites

https://exploringvolunteering.wordpress.com/author/paddaniels

On his 'Exploring volunteering' website Patrick Daniels has a very good page outlining the issues around professional values.

http://www.6cs.england.nhs.uk/pg/dashboard

The 6 Cs – the home site of the Compassion in Practice initiative.

Chapter 3
Communication

NMC Standards for Pre-registration Nursing Education

This chapter will address the following competencies:

Domain 1: Professional values

2. All nurses must practise in a holistic, non-judgemental, caring and sensitive manner that avoids assumptions; supports social inclusion; recognises and respects individual choice; and acknowledges diversity. Where necessary, they must challenge inequality, discrimination and exclusion from access to care.

Domain 2: Communication and interpersonal skills

1. All nurses must build partnerships and therapeutic relationships through safe, effective and non-discriminatory communication. They must take account of individual differences, capabilities and needs.

2. All nurses must use a range of communication skills and technologies to support person-centred care and enhance quality and safety. They must ensure people receive all the information they need in a language and manner that allows them to make informed choices and share decision making. They must recognise when language interpretation or other communication support is needed and know how to obtain it.

3. All nurses must use the full range of communication methods, including verbal, non-verbal and written, to acquire, interpret and record their knowledge and understanding of people's needs. They must be aware of their own values and beliefs and the impact this may have on their communication with others. They must take account of the many different ways in which people communicate and how these may be influenced by ill health, disability and other factors, and be able to recognise and respond effectively when a person finds it hard to communicate.

Chapter aims

After reading this chapter, you will be able to:

- outline the fundamentals of verbal and non-verbal communication;
- understand perception, the creation of 'self', and the impact of impression management on communication;

- understand what is meant by stigma and describe how labelling can affect a person's care;
- begin to explore how technological developments affect healthcare.

Introduction

Communication is a large topic, covered in detail in other books (e.g. Bach and Grant, 2015), but this chapter gives an introduction to the subject specifically in relation to psychology and sociology. A key message is that communication is a complex process which we often find ourselves poorly equipped to navigate. It is therefore just as important to try to understand ourselves as to understand others. It should also be remembered that communication involves at least two people, and that the person giving a message and the one receiving it may understand that message very differently. A point that has been continually stressed in the literature is that both verbal and non-verbal communication are to a considerable extent learned rather than being instinctive. This is demonstrated by the fact that they differ from language to language and from culture to culture (Lyons, 1977).

The chapter begins by examining the fundamentals of verbal and non-verbal communication, and then looks at some ideas around perception and self. This is because communicating with others involves how we perceive ourselves and how we perceive others. We will also explore Goffman's (1963) notion of stigma in an attempt to understand how perception shapes patient experiences. We will introduce labelling theory and how this might shape our behaviour and perceptions about people. New communication technologies will also affect nursing practice and we need to understand a little of how this impacts on how we define our work as well as the effects on patients.

Verbal communication

Verbal communication, of course, uses words which are units of speech or writing. Native speakers usually regard words as the smallest meaningful units of a language. They thus act as units of meaning. Words combine to convey an infinite variety of meanings. Words can be:

- precise;
- unambiguous;
- analytical – that is, they can break down concepts.

In scientific and analytical work we try to apply this in our language, but not always successfully. Consider what the word 'nursing' means to the public and what nursing theorists such as Nancy Roper may mean by the same word (Roper et al., 2000). In normal conversation, however, we only say things that we believe will be new to the listener. This is the 'given-new' contract in which speakers make assumptions about what the listener already knows.

This can be a problem for students who, when writing, do not say things that are 'obvious' and therefore do not get the marks they think they deserve. More importantly, it may be a problem when people, e.g. nurses, make assumptions about what their audience, i.e. patients, knows. For example, nurses know the internal anatomy whereas the lay public may not, so when we talk about organs and illness many patients will have little idea of what we are talking about. This is also complicated by mental health issues such as social anxiety disorder (social phobia), which is a persistent fear about social situations. It is much more than just 'shyness'; it causes intense, overwhelming fear over what may just be an everyday activity like shopping or speaking on the phone, or attending an outpatients clinic. People affected by it may fear doing or saying something they think will be humiliating. In addition, nurses may understand that what looks like 'social phobia' may be a result of either voices in one's head or feelings of lack of self-worth. The patient may just experience particular symptoms and may not know what social phobia means.

Verbal communication, then, is fraught with traps for the unwary, and of course the game of 'Chinese whispers' exploits human frailty in giving and receiving verbal communication.

Questions

Nurses, when assessing and undertaking patient consultations, will use questions which may be open or closed. Open questions:

- elicit more information;
- are more likely to lead to spontaneously given information;
- require more effort from the respondent.

An example of an open question might be: 'Tell me how you are feeling today' rather than the closed question, 'Are you well?'

Closed questions should be used if:

- simple factual information is needed;
- the respondent does not have the capacity to respond to open questions.

For example: 'What is your date of birth?' is a closed question, generating simple, factual information.

Words and their associations

Words can have force, they can hurt, and they can have hidden meanings that may convey particular, sometimes negative, messages to people. We should consider avoiding potentially stigmatising terms. For example:

- Use the phrase, 'He is a person with schizophrenia', rather than 'He is a schizophrenic'.
- 'She is a wheelchair user' is the acceptable term, rather than 'She is wheelchair-bound'.
- Find positive expressions. For example, a condom manufacturer describes the three sizes it produces as 'large', 'medium' and 'trim'.

We should not underestimate the power words may have, particularly if they carry within them a long-established negative connotation. None of us likes being sworn at, and words such as bastard, loony or spastic, or racially abusive words can wound at several different levels, recalling as they do a negative cultural mind set towards whole groups in society. Children may well be sensitive to the words used about them. Words constantly used by significant adults in their lives can be internalised by children, and therefore contribute to the building of their own ideas about themselves and of who they are. Gerhardt (2010a) alludes to this process, focusing on the early years of 0–3 as crucial in healthy child psychological and physical development.

Non-verbal communication

Non-verbal communication has a number of roles. It runs parallel to verbal communication and is often unconscious and may be ambiguous. It supports verbal communication, e.g. in turn taking, and of course is an alternative to verbal communication when verbal communication is not possible. It involves the following forms:

- facial expression;
- gaze;
- gestures;
- posture;
- proximity, i.e. how close we get to each other.

Paralanguage

Paralinguistics are the non-verbal means people use to convey meaning and emotion. Paralanguage involves:

- tone;
- intonation;
- pace;
- volume;
- accent.

Activity 3.1   *Communication*

Imagine that you are ringing a friend and that you get a wrong number. What you hear is the phrase, 'Hello, Sarah here'. What might paralinguistics tell you about Sarah? Experiment with different ways of saying the phrase to convey different messages about Sarah.

Can you give examples of non-verbal 'leakage' where non-verbal messages are accidentally conveyed?

An outline answer to this activity is given at the end of the chapter.

We engage in regulating our conversations. To do this, we signal the end of an utterance by looking up at the listener. Listeners signal that they are about to speak by looking away. Listeners signal interest by nodding, non-verbal noises, by looking at the speaker and by postural echo. Listeners can signal lack of interest by not doing these things. Not all of our communication is thus under conscious control, although we think we are in control of how we come across. The elements we have control over may start with facial expressions, then in descending order of control are our paralanguage, posture and limb movements: people are often not aware of foot tapping or movement.

We also use proximity – you know when someone invades your personal space – and eye contact to communicate either warmth or hostility. One issue to note here is that the distance involved in personal space varies between cultures. North Americans are said to prefer more distance than South Americans. As a nurse, you will often have to move into the personal space of others. Warn them when you are going to do this and tell them why it is necessary. Reduce eye contact while close to reduce the intensity of communication.

Non-verbal communication is affected by our cultural background, which we need to attend to if we are not to misread messages. Aspects to look out for include eye contact, interpersonal space, physical contact, smiling and the readiness to display emotion. Cultural competence (Helman, 2007) as an idea has arisen because of the diversity of cultural and ethnic groupings, especially in the USA, but of course it is also relevant in many metropolitan areas of the UK. The idea of cultural competence is to improve communication with minority and immigrant groups. Leininger (1995) has developed this idea into the concept of 'transcultural nursing', which emphasises the need to be sensitive to differences in values, beliefs, communication and practices. For example, in the Chinese community many will look to the ground when greeting someone, and it is considered disrespectful to stare into another person's eyes. Frowning while someone is speaking is a sign of disagreement, so many Chinese maintain an impassive face when speaking. This may appear uncomfortable to the untutored Western eye. As China is a large country there are regional variations, which makes things more complicated. However, a common posture is lowering of head and bending slightly to show respect, especially to an older person.

Remember also that disability can mean that a person cannot make the normal movements of non-verbal communication; for example, Parkinson's disease can reduce facial expression. It may also prevent the assumption of the expected postures and interfere with expected paralinguistic cues. Problems with sight or hearing can prevent a person from perceiving the incoming messages correctly, making it difficult to respond.

Children

Communication with children is another field altogether as the various stages of cognitive, physical and emotional development have to be taken into account. Children's understanding and their production of language and non-verbal communication will, of course, be different from those of an adult. It is all too easy to misunderstand a child's expressed needs and wants. Parents may be able to act as translators for a young child; however, it may be worth getting to know the child because a key factor in communication is the relationship and trust between adult and child. When it is possible, an investment in establishing a relationship will bring dividends.

Children understand and believe non-verbal communication, so ensure that your non-verbal communication and speech are congruent. The best way of calming a child may be to ensure the parent understands what is happening and is reassured, because relaxed parents communicate relaxation to the child.

(For further reading on this, see *Psychological Care in Nursing Practice*, by Michael Hyland and Morag Donaldson (1989), which has an excellent section on caring for children.)

Young children may see illnesses as all being contagious, which may mean they are afraid of proximity to any illness; or they may see illness as being a punishment, which may mean that they feel guilty about being ill or in pain. If they understand the actual cause, this will reduce the feelings of fear or guilt. Reassurance may be necessary in order to allay unnecessary fears built on incomplete understanding. The understanding of illness will become more sophisticated as the child gets older, with many 11-year-olds having a fairly good understanding of health and illness. (See Chapter 8 for more about nursing children.)

Activity 3.2   *Reflection*

- Try to notice your own use of language and non-verbal communication.
- Reflect upon how people react to your language and non-verbal communication.
- Notice other people's communication and reflect on how it makes you feel.
- Practise listening carefully, both to what people say to you, and to the feeling behind the message.

As this activity will be based on your own experience and reflections, there is no outline answer at the end of the chapter.

Guidance from the NHS

A useful source for information, including links to other organisations, can be found on NHS Choices: **http://www.nhs.uk/CarersDirect/guide/communication/Pages/Communicating. aspx**. This page points you to sources of support for those with communication difficulties.

The Aiding Communication in Education Centre offers help and support for children who have complex physical and communication difficulties, and for their parents, carers or therapists (**http://acecentre.org.uk**).

The charity I Can works to foster the development of speech, language and communication skills. They have a special focus on children with a communication disability (**www.ican.org.uk**).

Perception

The sociopsychology of perception involves understanding many ideas and concepts which are discussed in depth in other books (see the further reading list at the end of this chapter). Key terms in the sociopsychology of perception include:

- self-image;
- self-esteem ideal;
- self social comparison;
- self-consciousness;
- self-fulfilling prophecy;
- simple biases in impression formation;
- halo effect;
- impression management;
- primacy and recency effect;
- stigma;
- stereotyping;
- prejudice;
- discrimination;
- attribution/attribution errors.

This section focuses on the perception of others and the self. Perception, the way we see and interpret the world, may be dependent on our genes, our experience and our behaviour (Chalmers, 1997). The study of illusions and ambiguities suggests that the brain is engaged in trying to make sense out of sensory input; that is, it tries to make order out of chaos.

We may infer that communication involves making sense of a great deal of sensory input (how someone looks, how a person speaks – even how someone smells!) and that in trying to get a message across or understanding a message there is a good deal of unconscious brain work going on. The brain is thus trying to make sense of complexity. As we shall see in Chapter 5 on decision making, the brain often takes short cuts and can be fooled by a variety of factors. This is why we so often get things wrong.

False perception

Gestalt psychology emphasises the brain's attempt to produce perception from a range of complex stimuli. It is often easier to demonstrate than to describe. For example, look at Figure 3.1.

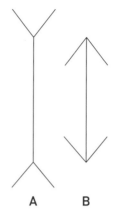

Figure 3.1: The Müller-Lyer illusion: Which line is longer, A or B?

Most people looking at the Müller-Lyer illusion think that A is longer. In fact, lines A and B are the same length.

In 1972, Richard Gregory proposed that perception is a series of guesses or hypotheses which are tested against previous experience, and then the nearest match is chosen. He explains the Müller-Lyer illusion in terms of the brain making mistakes about the relative depths of the two lines because we apply the rules that apply to three-dimensional perception to two-dimensional images. Thus, in the three-dimensional real world similar objects are judged to be the same size whether viewed close up or at a distance. We are used to seeing outside corners of buildings with lines sloping inwards away from them. In these situations, the brain knows that the line running down the outside corner is the closest part of the image to us. The brain realises that this line is really shorter than it appears when compared to the rest of the building.

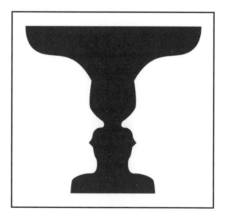

Figure 3.2: The face–vase illusion: Is it two faces or is it a vase?

The face–vase was devised by Edgar Rubin around 1915. It has become famous as an illustration of how humans construct an understanding of the world. It is suggested that we focus on figures within the visual field and the background surrounding any figures in order to gain appreciation of depth. The picture in Figure 3.2 is only two-dimensional but we fill in the gaps and perceive it as three-dimensional. In the case of the face–vase illusion, two ambiguous figures compete with an uncertain background for dominance within the visual centres. We therefore perceive alternating vase and faces, but can never perceive faces and vase simultaneously.

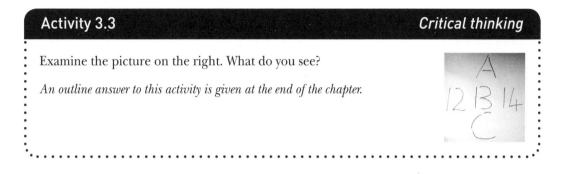

Activity 3.3 — *Critical thinking*

Examine the picture on the right. What do you see?

An outline answer to this activity is given at the end of the chapter.

Perception: construction and impression management

Consider the following and note that the brain works to make sense of the sentences using *constructs* that we are familiar with to make sense of disorder:

> *Pyscholgists tihnk taht prepsetoin is a contsurtive porcess wtih indviudals mkaing snese of snetneces by intreprteing rlues and aplpynig tetm to a contxet. Porviding the nmuber of lteters is corerct and the frist and lsat letetrs are in the rihgt odrer the snetence can be unedrstood.*

So, if the brain is using rules we are dimly aware of to make sense out of the physical world, is it doing the same with understanding people and communication? Fiske (2004) suggests that this may be the case, that we are actually using a *psychological lens* which helps us to see and interpret the person before us. We use processes of *selection, organisation* and *inference.*

We may *select* an aspect of a person's behaviour or appearance, and then try to form a coherent picture of who that person is by *organising* the data we have and then making *inferences* about that person based on the understanding.

A client shouts at us. This then is *selected* as an aspect of that person. The data we have about that person (just by looking at him) is that he is dressed in a dishevelled manner, his hair is unkempt and that his eyes are wide open and staring. We try to organise that data. Do these aspects fit a picture we have come across before? For example, can I see other clues (do his clothes smell?) that fit this into a coherent picture (this person looks like he lives on the streets – maybe this person is homeless?). Then we may infer from this that this person may have mental health problems (or has been drinking) and this is the reason for the shouting.

Of course, these inferences can be completely flawed. There could be more than one explanation for what we think we are seeing. The professional will suspend judgement until there is more evidence to be assessed.

Except that we don't always suspend judgement at all – professional nurses are still using human psychological constructs of selection, organisation and inference. Stockwell's (1972) description of the *unpopular patient* and nurses' reactions to perceived deviant behaviour suggested that nurses did not act non-judgementally to patients; that in fact they acted upon a variety of verbal and non-verbal cues to make inferences. In 1979 Jeffery described moral evaluations made by staff on the behaviour and presentation of patients in casualty departments, labelling some as *normal rubbish.*

Johnson and Webb (1995) later argued that social judgements and moral evaluations are not tied to the traits or characteristics that patients actually hold, such as diagnostic label or biographical details. Evaluations are also socially constructed by ward staff within social influences. Power, status and uncertainty are part of that evaluative process which ends up with patients labelled as 'good/ bad' or 'popular/unpopular'. Their study publicised the following phrases heard on the ward:

- 'He's a lovely man.'
- 'Oh, he's a right one.'

But they argue that such labelling occurs in social contexts and these are not necessarily actual traits 'possessed' by patients; rather they arise because of interaction, moral evaluation and judgement. Katz and Alegria (2003) seem to be making the same point about judgements and assumptions, this time in a US context within diagnostic interviews.

There is little reason to believe that clinicians have stopped 'selecting, organising and inferring' and making moral evaluations and social judgements about patients in a communicative encounter at the bedside or anywhere else. Indeed, Hill (2010), in his discussion of moral judgement, argued that it is *pervasive . . . [and] functions via a complex calculus that reflects variation in patient characteristics, clinician characteristics, task and organisational factors.* In other words, the setting, the task in hand, and type of people patients and clinicians are all impact on how we go about making moral evaluations of our patients. This demonstrates both social and psychological processes at work in our communications with patients.

Erving Goffman wrote *The Presentation of Self in Everyday Life* in 1959, using the metaphor of a theatre to discuss our everyday human interaction. He introduced the concept of *dramaturgical analysis* and argued that we play out interactions as if on stage. We have 'fronts' as part of our 'impression management' in our attempts to control what others may think of us.

Managing impressions is a two-way process. No doubt we wish to manipulate the inferences people make about us by emphasising certain characteristics so that we give the most positive impression we can. Our uniform (if we wear one) is an important aspect of impression management. The stethoscope around the neck gives out clues. Illness, of course, hinders impression management in that we lose control over the selection processes and the data we 'give off' is not in our control. Being in acute pain severely hampers our ability to communicate who we are.

Roper et al.'s (2000) model of nursing discusses *expressing sexuality* as an important activity of daily living. This implicitly acknowledges how we need to undertake certain practices (e.g. makeup for females, shaving for males) to present ourselves (impression management) to the world in an acceptable manner both to ourselves and to others. There is also a suggestion that first and last impressions count (*the primacy and recency effect*). If that first impression is one of 'likeability', or physical attractiveness, this forms a *halo,* which results in other favourable characteristics being attributed to that person (even if there is no evidence that the person has those positive characteristics). The reverse may also be true. Celebrity endorsements of products exploit the positive halo effect to sell goods and services.

These, often unconscious, processes affect how we go about communicating with people. The process of putting over a good impression is a way of communicating something about who you are and how you wish to be treated and spoken to. You are attempting to get value and be valued through this process. We have already noted that professionals put a certain value upon themselves and what they know, and that this then communicates itself to patients. If this is uncritical and unconscious, then certain unvoiced assumptions ('I know best because I know how this system works and I am educated') will come through in your unconscious impression management of your self. You will then alter how you are perceived.

Activity 3.4   *Reflection*

List the practical activities you undertake to prepare yourself before you leave the house in the morning.

Consider how these may be affected and changed by where you are going and who you plan to meet.

Think about the ways in which inpatients lose control of their ability to manage impressions. How might this affect their interaction with staff?

As this activity will be based on your own experience and reflections, there is no outline answer at the end of the chapter.

Self

The sense of who we are (self) is an important concept in healthcare. In order for us to be effective caregivers, we need to have some self-awareness. The perception of who we are may influence the way that we relate to those under our care. It is not just our own sense of self that is important. Patients'/clients' sense of self can often be affected by illnesses, or difficult experiences which they encounter. The way we understand these changes may lead us into responding in a helpful (empathetic) or unhelpful (prejudiced, discriminatory) manner.

This suggests that nursing work is not only about caring 'for' patients but is also an intensely psychosocial activity that creates the nurse's sense of self, perhaps also creating a 'professional identity'. The theory of social/professional identity suggests that a shared knowledge base and thus a shared professional language lead to shared identity. If groups identify and value themselves through various means, including using a particular language, it could be argued that in certain care settings, e.g. critical care, where medical and nursing knowledge overlaps and the language becomes commonly understood and used, there may be a basis for respect and value between the professions. In this manner, one 'becomes' identified as 'critical care nurse'. Willetts and Clarke (2014) outline the key concepts in social identity theory, which they use to address professional identity. They emphasise the daily activities of nurses in certain clinical contexts as the foundations for understanding the professional identity, and I would argue a sense of self, for nurses.

This links to discussions around 'values' and the '6Cs for compassionate practice' (Department of Health, 2012b). These are contextual arguments for developing cultures of care and imply that nurses can 'create themselves' using these values to be who they are. It might be hoped that, if clinical cultures expressly adopt and discuss the 6Cs, then they become part of the professional identity of the nurse. Whether that hope can be realised in actual practice is another matter.

Concept summary: The 'looking-glass self'

The *looking-glass self* (Cooley, 1902) happens when someone gets an idea of him- or herself based on other people's perceptions. This idea then leads the person to behave in a way that reinforces those perceptions.

There are three main components of the looking-glass self (Yeung and Martin, 2003):

- We imagine how we must appear to others.
- We imagine the judgement of that appearance.
- We develop our self through the judgements of others.

So consider these questions:

- What labels were put on you as you grew up and what effect did they have on you?
- What labels would you like to have now?
- What labels would you like to avoid now?
- What effect would these labels have on the way you see yourself?

Then consider the following:

- What labels would patients like to have?
- What labels would patients like to avoid?
- How would these labels affect the way the patient sees himself or herself?

  1. in helpful ways;
  2. in unhelpful ways.

Do labels affect the way you relate to others?

Are there any differences between how you relate to your peers, superiors, or someone subordinate to you?

Self-attribution bias

We may consider ourselves rational people who can work out who we are based on clear reasoning and evidence. However, we are prone to biases in thinking that we may not be aware of. It may also be the case that, even if we are aware of these errors in thinking, we still keep on making the errors. We constantly fall into using 'errors of thinking' or cognitive biases.

George Monbiot (2011) gave an interesting example of a 'cognitive bias' – the 'self-attribution' fallacy. He used the work of Daniel Kahneman, which he suggested is *devastating* to the beliefs that men who work in the City of London's financial district have about themselves. He argued that their apparent success is a cognitive illusion. He studied the results achieved by 25 financial advisers such as hedge fund managers across 8 years. He found that the consistency of their performance was zero. *The results resembled what you would expect from a dice-rolling contest, not a game of skill. Those who received the biggest bonuses had simply got lucky* (Monbiot, 2011).

Such results have been widely replicated. They show that traders and fund managers across Wall Street receive their massive remuneration for doing no better than would a chimpanzee flipping a coin. When Kahneman tried to point this out, they blanked him. *The illusion of skill . . . is deeply ingrained in their culture* (Monbiot, 2011). So a false sense of self builds up, one may suggest by reinforcement by colleagues and selective interpretation of actual events through the process of the 'looking-glass self'.

Fundamental attribution error

Fundamental attribution error (also known as *correspondence bias* or *attribution effect*) describes the tendency to give undue emphasis to personality-based explanations for the observed behaviour of others while undervaluing explanations based on the situation for those behaviours. The fundamental attribution error is most visible when people explain the behaviour of others. It is not usually used by people to explain their interpretations of their own behaviour. Situational factors are more likely to be taken into consideration in those cases. This discrepancy is called the actor–observer bias.

For example, if staff nurse Jacky saw staff nurse Brian making a drug error, Jacky might think that it is because Brian is careless (dispositional). If Jacky made the same error herself, she would be more likely to blame work stress or time constraints (situational).

So is it the person or is it the situation? Attribution error points us in the direction of blaming the person rather than the situation in which they find him- or herself.

Activity 3.5   *Critical thinking and reflection*

Choose a newspaper article regarding the report of a crime (e.g. the London lootings of summer 2011) which you think has portrayed those involved (either the victim(s) and/or perpetrator(s)) in a discriminative manner. Can you identify the reasons for this based on the attribution bias? Are there any stigma/stereotyping influences?

Have you ever suffered discrimination because of gender, race or other factors? How has this experience affected the way you see yourself, initially and afterwards?

An outline answer to this activity is given at the end of the chapter.

> **Scenario**
>
> *Mrs Smith, thin and emaciated, has taken an overdose of paracetamol. She has signs of multiple injection sites on her body and is now in accident and emergency (A&E). She has been seen by a nurse; she told the nurse that she was supposed to be taking medication for 'her condition' but had not taken the drug. The nurse has decided Mrs Smith's need is not urgent and so Mrs Smith is now waiting while more urgent cases are dealt with. Mrs Smith keeps calling out to staff as they pass, asking when she will see a doctor.*

If the above scenario had taken place while you were on placement in A&E, how might you have reacted, and why? In what ways has Mrs Smith's ability to manage her impression positively been compromised?

This may be a good time for you to pause and reflect on any stereotypes you hold. You might like to think about your perceptions of the characteristics of older people, younger people, people of other races, people with different sexual preferences from your own, males or females. If you feel uncomfortable doing this for any group, that is worth thinking about.

Would you be comfortable sharing your perceptions with somebody who belonged to that group? If not, why not?

As a general rule, the fewer members you know of a group, the more difficult it will be for you to respond to the individuality of the people within that group. However, remember that many of us hold stereotypical views of members of the opposite sex.

Stigma

The form communication should take means avoiding judgements based on stereotypes and labels. An important idea discussed in the literature is that of 'stigma', which draws us to the work of Erving Goffman (1963). The following fictional account outlines some of his key ideas. Words in **bold** are drawn from his work.

> **Scenario: Stigma – a narrative**
>
> *'Hello, my name is John and I am an alcoholic.'*
>
> *John (aged 46) lives alone in a bedsit in a less than salubrious part of town. He looks in the mirror each morning and thinks to himself – nothing. He just feels numb. Divorced, he does not know where his children are, and is now isolated as his employer reckons he can 'do without his services'. His previous landlord had given him notice to quit about 3 months ago.*

The landlord had stated at that time that John was not quite what he expected; his demeanour and appearance had deteriorated from when he first moved in. As he put it, John had 'undesired different-ness from what I had anticipated when I first took him in as a tenant'.

*John had carried his few belongings to the new place, feeling that now, as far as anyone else was concerned, he was reduced from a whole and usual person to a **tainted**, **discounted** one.*

*John is a drinker. When drunk, his alcoholism is out there for all to see – it has become a visible **discrediting** condition. Those around him can see and avoid him. In the mornings before his first drink he carries his alcoholism inside. He used to be able to function at work quite well, as his drinking was invisible, known only to himself (if he thought about it) as a **discreditable** condition that he was able to **pass** off.*

*Throughout his life he has struggled with feelings of self-hate and worthlessness. The drink was a friend. However, he knows it is not the friend it once was. He **feels** different, unwanted, alone. As life got more difficult, he could see the stares of strangers unless he was blind drunk. Being turned down for jobs and housing when his condition became known was increasingly hard to take. Employers and landlords saw him and **acted** according to the label 'alcoholic'. His wife eventually left him, unable to take the shame of having a drunk husband turn up at parties making a fool of himself. She had the **courtesy** of feeling the shame on his behalf.*

*It is not as if he had visible skin disfigurements or limbs missing (what some have called **abominations of the body**) – this is not why he felt different. After all, when sober, he had been fairly well presented and in his younger years quite a good-looking man. No, the issue now is that others think of him as weak, unable to control himself, a laughable character, with a **character blemish.** It is all to do with who he was as a person, not his family's fault – and he could not even argue he faced ethnic discrimination, living as he did among his own 'tribe'.*

*He feels socially worthless, and that the life he now lives is his fault. He is seen as **responsible** for his drinking. If he could just put the booze down, things could be better. However, some had seen him get worse over the years and thought there was nothing that could be done; the drinking was **progressively** worse and possibly **incurable**. Many friends and work colleagues had, of course, heard about alcoholism and many had drinking habits of their own which might be problematic. However, few had really **understood** what alcoholism actually was, how it arises, how it affects people, beyond seeing the drunk. And, of course, being drunk is often hard to **conceal**.*

John sits among the group feeling shame for his past behaviour and a little concerned about how this group might judge him. He has had enough experience of how other people have treated him recently and so feels apprehensive about the value judgements they would make and actions that this group might take. He is new to AA and has no idea how it works. He hopes that as the others have been (or still are) drinkers then maybe they would not judge him so.

*John's illness experience was being constructed in quite a negative way. His appearance and behaviour singled him out as **socially deviant**, subject to **discrimination**, **prejudice** and **stereotyping**.*

*His alcoholism was a condition of **societal deviance**, as most people accepted that this was a personal failing, a sign of moral weakness and lack of control. This was only slightly ameliorated by it also being seen as a disease. However, John's experience was not that of a patient with an illness that needs medical care; he felt outcast, alone and dirty. It was as if society had two definitions: alcoholism as disease, for which John should play the **sick role**, and alcoholism as deviant behaviour that requires punishment or avoidance.*

*John thus felt stigmatised: ostracised, devalued, rejected, scorned and shunned. He experienced discrimination, and only thinly disguised insults. He began to experience psychological distress, expressing **suicidal ideation** as a result of viewing himself with contempt. The drink paradoxically made that feeling go away. It was both saviour and nemesis.*

Activity 3.6   *Critical thinking and reflection*

Having read John's narrative, consider how stigma might form nurses' attitudes. What precautions can we take to prevent this? Nurses are people. People stigmatise based on cultural assumptions, values and experiences. Nurses are no different in this social process. However, critical reflective practice on a patient encounter may be a necessary step in uncovering our own value systems. To begin with, consider the following:

- a foul-mouthed drunk;
- a heroin user looking gaunt;
- a 14-year-old mother;
- a man who is obese and unshaven, with tattoos.

Consider the feelings that arise within yourself, and consider the picture you have in your mind's eye. What are your gut feelings towards these images? Where do these feelings come from, what are they based on and what is missing from your understanding?

Would the application of the sociological imagination and detailed background information on their life situations assist with untangling truth from prejudicial reality?

An outline answer to this activity is given at the end of the chapter.

Where does stigma come from?

Not everyone is comfortable with the term *stigma* or its connotations (Charlton, 1998). Critics have argued that stigma focuses too much on the characteristics of the stigmatised, and not enough on the *social and structural mechanisms* that create discrimination and entrench social oppression. So, for example, disabled people, or those with a mental illness, may become poor because they are excluded from decent employment as well as because of stigmatising attitudes.

Focusing on felt stigma diverts us from asking questions about issues of exclusion from society, which is a structural question. The criticism here is that efforts should be directed at understanding why society excludes people from decent work in these ways.

Thus, alcoholics can be stigmatised, but we have to ask ourselves *why* this is so. People with mental illness may experience stigma but again, *why* is this so? To understand their experience fully we have to examine the structures of society and the inner workings of our minds.

Should we be surprised at the number of people who have drink problems when we live in a society that actively promotes drinking as a social good, when just about all our social rituals have alcohol at their core, when so much ordinary social life is predicated upon drinking, when alcohol per unit is very cheap? This is the 'pull side' of alcohol, i.e. those aspects of social life that attract people to using drink. The 'push side' includes everyday problems with living: difficult personal relationships, work pressures and financial worries.

Returning to the ideas of C. Wright Mills (1959), to what extent is alcoholism a *personal trouble* only? To what extent is it also a *public issue?* What social structures are involved in 'creating' this as a personal and social problem?

What changes in society are implicated in problems with alcohol for individuals? What is occurring in the twenty-first century in certain societies that frames the alcoholic experience in particular ways?

We also need to consider the ways in which we discuss issues. What *discourses* are used to describe alcoholism – biomedical, psychiatric, criminal justice, public health, social? How does each discourse frame the issue? Is there a *nursing discourse* on alcoholism?

Concept summary: Stigma

Stigma may be an *undesired different-ness from what we had anticipated* (Goffman, 1963).

The stigmatised will be *reduced in our minds from a whole and usual person to a tainted, discounted one.*

1. Medical conditions which give rise to stigma can be:

   - discrediting conditions (visible), for example, psoriasis;
   - discreditable conditions (invisible), for example, HIV.

2. The experience of stigma can be:

   - felt – your subjective experience;
   - enacted – when discrimination takes place, moral judgements are made;
   - courtesy – when friends and family are involved and feel the discrimination or stigma.

3. Sources can include:

- 'abominations' of the body;
- blemishes of character, weak will, domineering or unnatural passions, treacherous and rigid beliefs, or dishonesty (blemishes of character are inferred from, for example, mental disorder, imprisonment, addiction, alcoholism, homosexuality, unemployment, suicidal attempts or radical political behaviour);
- tribal beliefs, e.g. arising from race, nation and religion (beliefs that are transmitted through lineages and equally contaminate all members of a family).

4. According to Goffman, diseases associated with the highest degree of stigma share common attributes.

- The person with the disease is seen as responsible for having the illness.
- The disease is progressive and incurable.
- The disease is not well understood among the public.
- The symptoms cannot be concealed.

See: Goffman, E (1963) *Stigma: Notes on the Management of Spoiled Identity*. Englewood Cliffs, NJ: Prentice Hall.

Note John's story above for an illustration of stigma in action.

Labelling theory

Howard Becker (1997) considered labelling in relation to deviant behaviour, and as we have noted, illness may be considered deviant from the norm of health. Deviance from the norm also includes those we label as alcoholics and drug addicts. The suggestion here is that there is no such thing as a deviant act. An act only becomes deviant when social actors define it as deviant. The example used is nudity, perfectly normal in one's marital bed but not so out in the street. There is nothing intrinsically deviant about nudity therefore.

Labelling, however, is applied to individuals and groups *by those who have the power* to make that label stick. These labels are then used to interpret behaviour as sick, normal, deviant, unpleasant. The behaviour may not have an intrinsic unpleasantness about it until the power group defines it as so, and they may do so based on the label they have put around the neck of the individual performing the act.

Activity 3.7   *Reflection*

Consider the labels of 'patient', 'client', 'doctor', 'nurse'. What meanings do we invest in these labels, and are there any implications for the roles people then play? Does a label make you feel different about yourself?

An outline answer to this activity is given at the end of the chapter.

The effects of labelling

A label is a value statement applied to the person who has the label.

- The label may become the *master status*, which overrides consideration of all other statuses and becomes the primary way in which one is seen and feels. The label 'diabetic' or 'schizophrenic', for example, may colour all other judgements and feelings. If there are negative associations with the label then this may be the way that people are considered and treated.
- *Self-fulfilling prophecy.* Your idea of who you are is drawn from how people see and treat you. Therefore, if you have a negative label (nutter, loony, schizo, druggy, wino) and this becomes your master status, you may see yourself as the nutter, loony, schizo, druggy, wino, and then adapt your behaviour to suit the label.

Stages in this process include the following.

- The individual is publicly labelled as deviant, followed by group rejection.
- Rejection encourages further deviance which prevents reintegration.
- The individual begins a *deviant career* as s/he cannot join straight society.
- The individual may join an organised deviant group as this is the only path to accepted identity.
- This develops into a deviant subculture which then begins to justify the lifestyle and supports deviant identity.

Deviance in common understanding may always have negative connotations, but what if deviance is merely deviance from the 'norm' and is thus merely *difference* – may this same process occur?

This idea supports notions of mental illness being to do with how we live our lives and the deviations in behaviour from that accepted norm. 'Madness' is thus merely deviation from the norm. Change the norms and the madness seems 'normal', or at least rational. We will return to this idea in Chapter 9.

Scenarios

Deviance as negative

Alan likes to bet, and his behaviour gets him the label 'gambler'. He loses so much money that he gets rejected from his work group and then his family. This label becomes his master status. Knowing this, he continues to gamble, thinking that the social harm has already been done. He then embarks on a gambling career as he is ostracised from society. He begins to hang out with other 'gamblers' in the casino and bookies, who don't judge him because of their own booze- and gambling-befuddled minds. He spends most of his time with fellow gamblers who all avoid any discussion about failures in family and work, and instead talk about anything that makes them feel good. Because he has now embraced the label of 'gambler', that is what he has now become, unable and/or unwilling to do anything about it.

continued . . . .

Deviance as neutral

Aisha feels unwell, gets tired easily, is thirsty and keeps passing urine. Her doctor tells her she is a 'diabetic'. Her family do not reject her but this new status brings attention and a focus on her needs that she has not experienced before. This becomes her master status. Accepting the label of 'diabetic', she throws herself into the role, finding out about diet and other issues which may become a challenge to her. Society does not reject her but she knows she is not 'normal' because she can't eat normal things and she thinks she has to plan activities around the fact of the diabetes. What she eats, what she drinks, what she feels she can do are all focused through the lens of diabetes. Sometimes she feels her husband does not understand how much she has to think about lifestyle changes. So she contacts other people with diabetes and joins an online support group.

Certain illnesses are not seen by society as (negatively) deviant but some may be (HIV, perhaps). Nonetheless, we may conclude that some diagnostic labels work for some people as a master status, colouring their judgement about themselves as well as how others may see them.

In the next section we discuss the increasing role technology has in communication. This is fast-paced development and hence it is foolish to predict what will be available to us in the next few years.

Communication technologies

As we are all well aware, the developments in information technologies are astounding, although those of you who are young enough to be what have been called 'digital natives', i.e. you have grown up in a world of computers and digital information as natural, may not be able to grasp fully the changes that have taken place. Information technology hardware has been transformed: smart phones, tablets and what the internet itself can now do in terms of interactivity, sharing and creativity are moving on at a very fast pace.

Technology is moving quickly to adapt to and adopt new innovations. Building on the increasing use of smart phones and tablet computers, there are now apps being developed for healthcare professionals to use in everyday clinical practice. The UK Resuscitation Council has its own app which allows easy access to the latest resuscitation guidelines (**https://play.google.com/store/apps/details?id=air.com.unit9.lifesaver.android.mobile**). There is now a website forum for commentary by medical professionals on medical app reviews (**www.imedicalapps.com**).

Technology in the workplace is part of everyday experience, but we need to think about how it is affecting who we are and how we communicate with each other. There is a question about whether technology affects the way we think.

Certain clinical situations make it critical that certain facts are brought to mind quickly and then acted upon. Knowing the facts of the clinical signs of hypovolaemic shock will save someone's life. Knowing *where* those facts are that outline the clinical signs of shock is not good enough if that 'where' is not in your head, as you may not have the time to check them out by referring to an app. How often do we need instant recall to save a life? Not that often, but rote-learning algorithms for basic life support cannot be delegated externally to, say, a server. However, the growing use of computers may be doing something to our memories and may be changing the way we are going about learning facts.

Betsy Sparrow and colleagues (2011) have studied the effects of Google on memory. They argue that when we are faced with complex problems we now begin to think about computers. This is because we know we can 'google' anything we want. The further effect this is having is that we have lower rates of recall. We don't remember the information itself; we remember *where* it is. The internet acts then as *transactive memory*, i.e. memory that is stored *externally* to ourselves. This relates to the idea of the 'group mind', whereby knowledge is shared among a group of individuals in an interdependent *cognitive* (knowledge) relationship. This may be seen in long-term relationships between two people who then rely on each other for memory.

If there is such a thing as a 'group mind' with transactive memory, then we may be seeing another facet of interprofessional working, and thus the need to evaluate carefully how we work together. Shared complex knowledge among a group of people in a *community of practice* (Wenger, 2000) may be a feature of working in clinical teams and therefore recognised as such.

Marshall McLuhan (1964) argued that *[t]he medium is the message. This is merely to say that the personal and social consequences of any medium – that is, of any extension of ourselves – result from the new scale that is introduced into our affairs* by any new technology. He went on to state: *[w]e shape our tools and afterwards our tools shape us.*

By that he means that, to understand new technologies, it is not the *content* that is so interesting; it is the effects that the technology has on thoughts, feelings, behaviours, cognitive and sociocultural practices, such as transactive memory. If Sparrow is correct, then the internet is shaping the way we store, retrieve and share memory beyond the obvious use of memory sticks, hard drives and iPhone apps such as Medscape.

Does this mean that the internet is now creating group memory and diminishing individual memory? Will the need to have individual facts in our own heads in the future diminish as the technologies develop? In addition, are students subconsciously not committing facts to memory because they know that the vast majority of what they require is available in 'the cloud'? As we have just stated above, tablet computers and smart phones are now bringing literally to your hand a store of knowledge that was just not available only a few years ago. The sheer weight of knowledge required for modern clinical practice may align with technological developments so that in future the key skill will be not *what* you know but *where* you know it.

More recent developments include the use of social media such as Twitter and Facebook requiring the development of 'digital professionalism'. Both media support educational activities such as at Plymouth University, where students have professional Twitter accounts as part of the educational process. New rules for communication have to be learned as these platforms were developed primarily for social rather than professional use. Schmitt et al. (2012) are generally positive in advocating their use in the education of nurses, as are Tuominen et al. (2014) in the context of Finnish nursing students' views.

At present the NHS is struggling with paper-based systems of communication, with difficulties arising from such day-to-day communication between hospitals and primary care and vice versa. Communication and information sharing within the NHS continues to be problematic. Fiona Caldicott chaired a review of NHS information systems and published a report called *Information to Share or not to Share: The Information Governance Review* (Department of Health, 2013). Issues arising from within the review included a lack of access to patient records by patients, resulting in 'great frustration'. A recommendation was that all letters, emails and other communication that teams make regarding patient care should be copied and made available for patients. Managers came under fire for being 'unduly restrictive' due to fears over data protection laws. Digital technologies have existed for quite a while but do not appear to be embedded into NHS communication systems sufficiently to prevent breakdown in communication.

Chapter summary

- Communication involves perception and the construction of self.
- Communication is a complex process, being verbal and non-verbal, including the use of paralinguistics.
- Stigmatising, labelling and stereotyping all affect communication, both in the way we process messages from other people and in the unspoken messages we convey back to them.
- Methods of communication are being affected in fundamental ways by technological developments, which in turn may affect our own thinking processes.

Activities: brief outline answers

Activity 3.1 Communication

If Sarah answers in a loud voice without hesitation, you might infer something about her self-confidence. If Sarah answers quietly and slowly draws the words out you might infer timidity.

An example of leakage could occur if someone who is asked out on a date says 'yes', but avoids eye contact and carries on with what they s/he was doing. Alternatively, if someone who is told of another's misfortune says, 'Oh, I am so sorry', while failing to keep a look of amusement from his or her face.

Activity 3.3 Critical thinking

When viewed from top to bottom, the symbol in the centre appears as the letter B. When viewed left to right, the same symbol appears as the number 13. Exactly the same symbol represents different things depending on context. Psychologists have studied the effect of illusions in order to examine how we perceive the world. They have concluded there is a difference between seeing and perceiving.

Activity 3.5 Critical thinking and reflection

David Cameron called the looters criminal *pure and simple*, thereby attributing the behaviour to personal deficiencies (dispositional – they had a *disposition* to be criminals). The London School of Economics report, however, suggested other factors might have been at work (e.g. police stop-and-search tactics).

These then are situational factors, that is to say, it was the situation the people experienced that encouraged that behaviour.

Activity 3.6 Critical thinking and reflection

In each case a feeling of superiority may arise towards the other due to ideas around personal moral failings that are based on their lack of education, their inability to take control of their lives, their deviant behaviour and ideas of 'low' culture (tattoos). What may be missing is their personal biographies, their stories, that led them to be where they are now. Was the drunk abused as a child? Was the 14-year-old abandoned by her parents? Was the obese man made unemployed (again)? How easy do you find it to modify your views when you understand more about the person's history and background?

Activity 3.7 Reflection

The label 'doctor' carries a very powerful social message and attracts prestige and status as well as remuneration at a high level. If you could put Dr in front of your name you would find many people will treat you differently, often with deference and respect. The reaction to the label 'nurse' may be that you are sexy, 'up for it', a self-sacrificing angel or just an uncaring abuser.

Further reading

Bach, S and Grant, A (2015) *Communication and Interpersonal Skills in Nursing*, 3rd edn. London: Sage/Learning Matters.

Goodman, B and Clemow, R (2010) *Nursing and Collaborative Practice.* Exeter: Learning Matters.

See Chapter 6 for a discussion on the psychological issues at play in interaction.

Gross, R and Kinnison, N (2007) *Psychology for Nurses and Allied Health Professionals.* London: Hodder Arnold.

Chapters 8 and 9 are key chapters on perception and attribution.

Haralambos, H and Holborn, M (2007) *Sociology Themes and Perspectives*, 7th edn. London: Collins.

For fuller discussions on stigma and labelling theory, see Chapter 6.

Useful websites

http://marshallmcluhan.com

If you want to investigate further how communication and media affect human relationships, then McLuhan is a very good starting point.

www.nwlink.com/~donclark/leader/leadcom.html

There are interesting resources on this site for communication and leadership – but don't let 'leadership' put you off. These may also be useful for later chapters.

http://www.nhs.uk/CarersDirect/guide/communication/Pages/Communicating.aspx

The NHS Choices site on communication advice for carers.

Chapter 4
Inequalities, social determinants of health and nursing practice

Chapter aims

After reading this chapter, you will be able to:

*   understand the arguments around the links between health and inequalities;
*   place health in a global context;
*   understand the role that 'discourse' has in providing explanations;
*   consider what this means for nursing practice.

Introduction

In the previous chapter we examined communication, noting how we need to understand our-selves as much as understanding others (Goodman and Clemow, 2010). This meant exploring ideas around the self and perception. Goffman's (1963) notion of stigma along with labelling theory may support understanding of how perceptions shape patient experiences. We also noted how new technologies of communication may begin to shape how we use our memories and change the way we work. In this chapter we will be exploring the relationship of psychology and sociology to nurs-ing practice. The other half of Domain 3, decision making, will be addressed in the next chapter.

Nursing practice, of course, means many things but for our purposes we will consider nursing practice as a *social activity* that takes place within the context of inequalities in health and the *social determinants of health approach* (World Health Organization, 2008). This balances the indi-vidual and biomedical focus of much of nursing practice, and which, in any case, is discussed at length in many other books.

Inequalities and the social determinants of health

Davidson (2015) outlines the origins of the social determinants of health approach, from the 1974 Lalonde Report in Canada to the Rio Declaration on the Social Determinants of Health signed in 2011. The Lalonde report endorsed Thomas McKeown's view that medical care and public health services played very little role in reducing illness and premature death (Davidson, 2015, p. 6). The premise is that biology and health services are relatively unimportant in com-parison to social factors.

The World Health Organization (2008) states:

> *The social determinants of health are the conditions in which people are born, grow, live, work and age. These circumstances are shaped by the distribution of money, power and resources at global, national and local levels. The social determinants of health are mostly responsible for health inequities – the unfair and avoidable differences in health status seen within and between countries.*

I think this introduces an ethical imperative and a sociopolitical role for nursing (Falk-Raphael, 2006), as the Nursing and Midwifery Council (NMC) explicitly states that nurses are to *work to improve health*. If health has social determinants based on the *distribution of money, power and resources* then nurses are required to understand what this means. Indeed, public health princi-ples are now embracing concepts such as the social determinants of health and going further in the ecological public health approach (Lang and Rayner, 2012). Understanding health also requires understanding politics as a key determinant of population health (Horton et al., 2014; Ottersen et al., 2014; Davidson, 2015).

So we need to consider the link between health inequalities and social inequalities and that health is not necessarily related to the provision of health services; it does however relate to issues around social class and material differences.

Scambler (2012) also suggests that the type and delivery of healthcare services are not decisive for health outcomes. Differential health outcomes, such as mortality and morbidity rates, are based in the conditions and experiences of everyday lives, and this shows a social gradient – the lower down on the socioeconomic scale you are, the worse your health outcomes. Scambler argues we must look to social class relationships as it is in class relationships that we see *asset flows* working in people's lives.

Scambler (2012) argues: *The noun 'flows' is significant here. People do not either have or not have assets positive for health and longevity, rather the strength of flow of these assets varies through the life-course.*

So it is not the static acquisition of wealth or material deprivation that is at work. It is about what assets flow in and out of people's lives over the course of their life, and this is particularly important in childhood and older age.

The 'assets' are:

- biological: your 'genetic inheritance', sex, your disabilities, your long-term conditions;
- psychological: your self-efficacy, locus of control, learned helplessness;
- social: your family network, community networks, friendships;
- cultural: your lifestyle choices, such as smoking, or ethnic background;
- spatial: where you live – leafy Surrey or inner-city Glasgow;
- symbolic: your status as a 'chav' or as member of the elite;
- material: your income and wealth.

It is important to stress that a strong flow of one asset can compensate for the weak flow of another. Scambler provides examples:

> *a strong psychological asset flow (i.e. high personal resilience) can cancel out the negative propensities of a weak flow of social assets (i.e. an absence of close-knit social networks); and a strong flow of symbolic assets (i.e. high social status) can mitigate the damage liable from a weak flow of spatial assets such as living in an area of deprivation.*

In addition, Scambler suggests that we need to understand that:

1. The strength of flow of material assets (i.e. standard of living via personal and household income) is paramount. This links with the material deprivation thesis, explaining the link between health inequalities and socioeconomic status.
2. Flows of assets tend to vary together (i.e. mostly strong or weak 'across the board').
3. Weak asset flows across the board tend at critical junctures of the life-course (e.g. during infancy and childhood) to have especially deleterious effects on lifetime health and longevity: a child born with a chronic illness, into the lowest decile of income distribution, in an abusive psychological and social environment, living in damp squalid housing in which both parents

smoke, in an area of high unemployment and poor access to healthcare and a proliferation of fast food outlets, in a culture that demonises 'chavs and benefits cheats'.

4. Weak asset flows across the board, and strong asset flows across the board, tend to exercise a cumulative effect over the life-course (negatively and positively, respectively); the 'subjective' evaluation of the strength of an asset flow can exert an effect over and above any 'objective' measure of that flow (e.g. a symbolic asset flow perceived as weak relative to that enjoyed by an individual's reference group can be injurious in its own right). That is, how we perceive how good or poor our 'asset' is affects us even if that asset is not in itself injurious. This is the social comparison thesis or psychosocial hypothesis.

Scambler regards the material asset flow as vital or *prepotent*. Of all assets it is the material conditions of life that underpin much of our health outcomes. To argue that material conditions underpin all other asset flows is not to diminish their importance for health inequalities. This is only highlighting the key point of Wilkinson and Pickett's (2010) *The Spirit Level*, in that action on the reduction in income inequality is a precondition for tackling health inequalities. Annandale and Field (2007) argue that inequalities in health between social groups are a resilient feature of British society. They also suggest that these inequalities will persist through the twenty-first century. Basu and Stuckler (2013) directly link inequalities, government policies, such as 'austerity', to illness and deaths. They argue that across Europe and North America 10,000 additional suicides and up to a million extra cases of depression have been recorded. They argue: *recessions hurt but Austerity kills.*

Danny Dorling (2014) points to the rising levels of inequality and argues that being born outside the 1 per cent per cent has a dramatic effect on a person's potential – that person's asset flows – reducing life expectancy, limiting educational and work prospects and adversely affecting mental health.

Scambler also suggests:

> *Our society, one in which income and health inequalities are rapidly rising, and in which policy . . . has allowed a Health and Social Care Act to deliver a proven cost-effective publicly owned NHS into the hands of transnational profiteers, is slipping into a post-welfare-statist, neo-liberal abyss.*

In other words, UK society is losing its NHS as it is being sold off piecemeal to private-sector providers who seek to make a profit, losing its welfare provisions, experiencing increasing social and economic divides, which are the *circumstances shaped by the distribution of money, power and resources* impacting on population health.

Finally, a nurse argues:

> *Considerable evidence suggests that neocolonialism, in the form of economic globalization as it has evolved since the 1980s, contributes significantly to the poverty and immense global burden of disease experienced by peoples of the developing world, as well as to escalating environmental degradation of alarming proportions. Nursing's fundamental responsibilities to promote health, prevent disease, and alleviate suffering call for the expression of caring for humanity and environment through political activism at local, national, and international levels to bring about reforms of the current global economic order.*
> (Falk-Raphael, 2006)

Inequalities of health can be seen both within and between countries, and hence exist on a global scale.

It is the case that there are very clear differences in health outcomes and access to disease care based on gender, ethnicity and socioeconomic position. This applies also to those with mental health problems and learning disabilities. There are several theories to account for these differences. However, understanding that health has *social determinants* (Marmot, 2010; Davidson, 2015) is a foundation to understanding the differences.

Global inequalities in health

In their book *The Spirit Level,* Wilkinson and Pickett (2010) argue that in developed societies there is a single root cause to almost every common social problem, i.e. reduced life expectancy, child mortality, drugs, crime, homicide rates, mental illness and obesity. That root cause is *inequality.*

Moreover, they claim, it is not just the 'deprived underclass' that loses out in an unequal society – everyone does, even those in higher socioeconomic groups. The reason for this is that it is not the *absolute* levels of poverty that create the social problems, but the *differentials* in income between rich and poor. Someone from the lowest-earning 20 per cent of a more equal society is more likely to live longer than a counterpart from a less equal society; so too, someone from the highest earning 20 per cent has a longer life expectancy than a counterpart in a less equal society.

The USA is wealthier and spends more on healthcare than any other country, yet a child born in Greece, where average income levels are about half that of the USA, has a lower risk of infant mortality and longer life expectancy than an American baby. Obesity is twice as common in the UK as in the more equal societies of Sweden and Norway, and six times more common in the USA than in Japan. Teenage birth rates are six times higher in the UK than in more equal societies; mental illness is three times as common in the USA as in Japan; murder rates are three times higher in more unequal countries. The examples in the book are numerous.

When extensive data became available from the World Bank in 2005, Wilkinson and Pickett realised that their focus of study – health is driven by relative difference rather than absolute material standards – applied in other areas of social policy. They noted that countries such as the USA, the UK and Portugal, where the top 20 per cent earn seven, eight or nine times more than the lowest 20 per cent, *scored noticeably higher on all social problems* at every level of society than countries such as Sweden and Japan, where the differential is only two or three times higher at the top.

To ensure their findings could not be explained by cultural differences, Wilkinson and Pickett analysed the data from all 50 US states and found the same pattern. In states where income differentials were greatest, so were the social problems and lack of cohesion.

Wilkinson and Pickett argue that the mechanism explaining the phenomenon is to be found in the psychosocial areas of hierarchy and status. The greater the differential between the haves and have-nots, the greater importance everyone places on the material aspects of consumption; what brand of car you drive carries far more meaning in a more hierarchical society than in a flatter one. It is the knock-on effect of this *status anxiety* that finds socially corrosive expression in crime, ill health and mistrust. While Wilkinson and Pickett's book has had a great deal of publicity and is based on a good deal of statistical evidence, the ideas presented in it have not been universally accepted and indeed have been critiqued (Snowdon, 2010). See useful websites at the end of this chapter on details of the Radio 4 *Analysis* broadcast.

Carlisle (2001) earlier argued that this inequalities debate is thus a contested issue, that there are differing conceptions of what the causes and solutions are to the identified problems and that there are at least three *discourses* which provide for people ways of knowing, thinking and talking about issues. These discourses do not always overlap and often are in conflict with each other. We will return to the notion of discourse below when we examine the work of Michel Foucault.

Activity 4.1   *Research and evidence-based practice*

Go to the United Nations' Millennium Development Goals (MDG) indicators home page: **http://mdgs.un.org/unsd/mdg/Default.aspx** and find the Data tag. Follow the link to Gapminder MDG chart. Browse the information, comparing things such as literacy rates. Also find and list the MDGs.

An outline answer to this activity is given at the end of the chapter.

How do we know a population is more or less healthy? There need to be a few indicators, health outcomes, that can be objectively measured. *Subjective* measures of well-being and 'happiness' are problematic for the purpose of comparison between populations. In addition, measures of subjective feelings of happiness take little heed of the social and material conditions in which people live and thus provide no basis for changing the sociopolitical conditions of people's lives.

Key objective measures of population health include the following:

- life expectancy;
- mortality statistics, particularly maternal, infant and child;
- morbidity statistics;
- employment;
- education (e.g. female literacy rates).

A systematic blueprint for objectively measuring and describing health and other development outcomes can be found in the United Nations 'project' which forms the MDGs.

Both within the UK and internationally, then, there is a recognition that in terms of health outcomes we live in a very unequal world. Activity 4.1 asks you to investigate the sheer scale of the issues. You will need to get a grasp of how *where* you were born, what *gender* you are, what *ethnic* group you belong to and crucially, what *socioeconomic status* your parents have affect your health outcomes. The issues are complex and there is discussion and debate about what the key determinants of health are. The answer for any one individual lies in the specific local contexts in which that person lives, that is, you need to investigate the social conditions as experienced in each person's case. For some people the main determinant for a specific health outcome is their gender; however, poverty, social exclusion and material deprivation have a great impact. In other words, it may be better to be born female in a wealthy developed country (e.g. Norway) than to be born male in a very poor country (e.g. Somalia) struggling to improve its health and education systems, and riven with civil unrest and very poor (if not totally absent) governance and security.

UK inequality

The following research summary illustrates some data showing the differentials in life expectancy for the UK, which indicate both a gender and a locality difference. There is a mass of data available showing differences for gender and ethnicity, as well as socioeconomic status. You can follow this up by accessing the useful websites at the end of this chapter.

Research summary: 'People in poor areas die younger'

The Office for National Statistics (ONS) found:

- In 2010–2012, male life expectancy at birth was highest in East Dorset (82.9 years) and lowest in Blackpool (74.0 years).
- For females, life expectancy at birth was highest in Purbeck, at 86.6 years, and lowest in Manchester, where females could expect to live for 79.5 years.
- On average, life expectancy at birth increased across all local areas in England and Wales by 1.3 years for males and 1.0 year for females between 2006–2008 and 2010–2012.
- Life expectancy at age 65 was highest for men in Harrow, where they could expect to live for a further 20.9 years compared with 15.8 years for men in Manchester.
- For women at age 65, life expectancy was highest in Camden (23.8 years) and lowest in Blaenau Gwent (18.7 years).
- The distribution of life expectancy across England was characterised by a north–south divide, with people in local areas in the north generally living shorter lives than those in the south.

In 2010–2012, approximately 28 per cent of local areas in the east, 49 per cent in the south-east and 28 per cent in the south-west were in the fifth of areas with the highest male life expectancy at birth. In contrast, there was no local area in the north-east and Wales in this group. A similar pattern was observed for females.

Go to the ONS website for full statistical information (**http://www.ons.gov.uk**). You can also look up data at the Institute of Health Equity (**http://www.instituteofhealthequity. org/presentations/presentation-slides**).

Now that we have established that disparities and inequalities in health exist, how do we account for them? We need to explore some explanations and important UK publications. But first we need to ask, what should be the response of nurses?

Activity 4.2   ***Critical thinking and team working***

Consider your position on the following question.

Do poverty and ill health arise from the failings of individuals or from failings of society?

Write some first thoughts on this question and share with colleagues.

Consider what evidence you have for your position: can you refer to any?

An outline answer to this activity is given at the end of the chapter.

Explanations for inequalities in health

The main explanations given for inequalities in health are as follows:

- Hereditarian explanations: everyone has a biologically determined natural capacity, thus little can be done (individualist explanation).
- Behavioural explanations: the lifestyle choices of individuals are the cause; the answer is education (or punishment).
- Environmental explanations: the cause is a person's social position and material deprivation, so the answer is structural.

So, explanations are either individualistic/behaviourist and/or structural/materialist.

Another way of expressing this is by talking about *contemporary explanations*, though there are overlaps between these explanations. A simplified typology is as follows.

- poverty/deprivation (structuralist/materialist – environmental);
- psychosocial stress (structuralist/materialist – environmental – behavioural);
- individual deficits (individualist/behavioural – hereditarian).

This is a live issue, because the solutions to inequalities in health depend on why you think they exist in the first place. Health policy derives from the positions that influential policy makers and lobbyists take. Underlying the explanations are what are known as 'discourses'. These are mental conceptions about how the world works involving personal theories, values and philosophies. Discourses are not always checked against evidence.

Health based on poverty and its measurement

One of the explanatory frameworks, or 'discourses', for ill health and health inequalities around access to health services and health outcomes, is that of the 'material deprivation' thesis mentioned above, which underpins much of the Marmot (2010) review, *Fair Society, Healthy Lives*. It sits within a 'redistribution discourse', which suggests the answer is redistribution of material resources. Alongside this is the 'psychosocial comparison thesis', which underpins work such as Wilkinson and Pickett's (2010) *The Spirit Level*. This forms part of the 'social integrationist discourse', in which reduction of social inequalities and better integration of marginalised groups are important.

Material deprivation (and latterly, neomaterialist) focuses on a lack of resources to support healthy living while psychosocial comparison suggests one's position in the social hierarchy, and the level of inequality in society, create psychosocial stress harmful to health. They are not mutually exclusive and, of course, might work together for some individuals, resulting in poorer health outcomes for them. Being poor in a very unequal society is thus very harmful to health and results in gross inequalities in health.

A third explanatory framework is the 'cultural thesis', which suggests it is the culture of certain behaviours, attitudes, values and norms that is the root cause of ill health. Another term for this way of thinking is the 'moral underclass discourse'. People should make better choices and improve lifestyle activities, such as stopping smoking, reducing alcohol consumption, exercising more and eating better. Poor people are disproportionately ill because of their poor life decisions. The 'underclass' make poor moral decisions and therefore bring ill health upon themselves. The material deprivation they experience is a result of their own poor life choices, their parents' life choices, or it results from being ill, preventing them from working or making better life choices (the deserving poor).

The consensual method of measuring poverty

A link between all three is material deprivation resulting from poverty, but what do we mean by poverty and how is it measured? In the UK we do not use the concept of absolute poverty; instead some reports are using the term 'relative poverty', one measure of which is the consensual method. The research project Poverty and Social Exclusion (PSE) outlines what this is (**http://www.poverty.org.uk/summary/social%20exclusion.shtml**). In short this focuses on deprivation as: *enforced lack of necessities determined by public opinion.*

In the consensual approach we first need to establish what those items are that make up our 'standard of living' and then identify which of those items most people view as 'necessities'. Consider a mobile phone as an item: if most people think this is a necessity, then not having one begins to identify oneself as poor. The necessities are what most people think everyone should be able to afford and which no one should be without. Poverty is where these deprivations impact on a person's whole way of life; to measure poverty we need to know how many people there are whose '*enforced* lack of necessities' affects their way of living. Note that those who choose not to have these necessities would not count.

Items that are necessary include the social as well as the material. The PSE has published data on what the public thinks those items are: for example, 96 per cent of us think 'heating to warm living areas of the home', 94 per cent think a 'damp-free home' and 91 per cent think 'two meals a day for adults' are some of the necessities. However some items go beyond 'basic' needs, such as 'visiting friends/family in hospital' (90 per cent), and 'attending a wedding/funeral' (79 per cent).

- What do you think *everyone* should be able to afford?
- What do you think no one should be without?

Once we have these benchmarks, then we can start to measure the baseline below which society considers people to be deprived. This is what has been attempted since 1983 and the *Breadline Britain* report (London Weekend Television, 1983).

The first PSE report, *The Impoverishment of the UK: PSE First Results – Living Standards* (Gordon et al., 2013), indicates the scale and extent of poverty in the UK – the sixth richest country as measured by gross domestic product per capita. One section of the report *Going Backwards 1983–2012* suggests that the proportion of households falling below minimum standards has doubled since 1983 (Poverty and Social Exclusion, 2013):

1. More children lead impoverished and restricted lives today than in 1999.
2. Five million more people live in inadequate housing than in the 1990s.
3. Nine per cent of households can't heat their homes adequately today, up from 5 per cent in 1983 and 3 per cent in 1999.
4. Thirty-three per cent of households experience below-par living standards.

This is despite the fact that the UK is a far richer country now than it was in the 1980s. The size of the economy has doubled over the last 30 years. This supports the claim that economic and wealth creation has benefited the better off while families lower down continue to struggle to meet their basic needs.

If you emphasise that ill health and deprivation result from poor life choices, i.e. you base your explanations in the cultural thesis, then you might not be interested that more and more families are experiencing deprivation of this kind. For you, it is a case of them not taking up opportunities, not changing bad cultural habits, not working hard at their education or not moving to where employment is higher. However, you might want to wonder why more and more families are making these poor life choices since the 1980s, especially if during that time knowledge about what is the basis for a healthy life is more easily accessible with the internet. This increasing pool of 'the underclass' who choose poor lifestyles and who cannot afford what the majority consider to be a decent lifestyle requires some explanation.

Or, you might think that, regardless of the fact that more people are falling into this category of deprivation, this does not mean that they are also more likely to experience health inequalities such as reductions in life expectancy. You may think that there is no link between living below minimum standards and poorer health outcomes. The answer is complicated. Mackenbach (2012) outlines nine 'theories' explaining health inequalities and argues there are at least three conditions that help to explain the persistence of health inequalities in modern welfare states: (1) material inequalities have not been eliminated; (2) the personal characteristics related to ill health of those in lower socioeconomic groups remain similar; and (3) the benefits of being in a higher social position have increased.

Discourse

French social theorist Michel Foucault developed a notion of *discourse* in his early work, especially *The Archaeology of Knowledge* (1969). Lessa (2006) summarises Foucault's definition of discourse as *systems of thoughts composed of ideas, attitudes, courses of action, beliefs and practices that **systematically construct the subjects** and the worlds of which they speak* (p. 283).

(The word 'subject' here refers to us as human 'subjects' – as in the *subjective* self. The world outside of ourselves is the object, the objective world.)

In other words, *a discourse* is a specific collection of words or phrases that have a particular meaning and in using a discourse we (*the subjects*) create (*construct*) the social world we are describing. For example, when a community uses the words 'loony, nutter or psycho' the world they create (in their heads) in using those words includes a category of people that are different, maybe a bit scary; certainly we don't quite understand them or why they are like they are, and we may feel the need to segregate them to protect ourselves from them.

This is the lay discourse that creates a certain picture of mental illness. It is constructing a certain world in which there are 'loonies'.

A community that uses the words 'bipolar disorder', 'problem with living' or 'depression' creates a world in which certain attitudinal and behavioural characteristics can be explained in terms of organic brain disease or poor cognitive and emotional functioning that require a range of therapies to address. This world has patients and clients instead of 'loonies'. This world may not be quite as frightening, as we have an idea of what the causes might be and hence what treatments might work. We seek to include these people into society in an attempt at 'cure' or rehabilitation.

Communities share discourses and that may act as a form of shorthand because the community 'knows' what is being said. Foucault goes further and suggests that discourse relates to the exercise of power in society, i.e. if a powerful group can get society to accept their discourse as the 'one true' discourse, then that gives a good deal of influence over how society then operates.

Consider an objective fact such as an explosion which kills a man in a soldier's uniform who is carrying a gun. What sense can we make of that incident? Is it a tragic death of a man fighting for freedom or is it a glorious death on the path to freedom from oppression? The 'war on terror' discourse sees it one way: he is a 'freedom fighter', one of 'our boys'. The Islamist jihad discourse sees it another way: he is an oppressor, an 'infidel'. Both discourses involve modes of speech ('our boys', 'infidel'), ideas and attitudes which then act to create a social world and a social meaning to their users.

In this extreme example it can be seen that two opposing discourses make it very difficult to come to a shared understanding of the incident, and very difficult to come to an agreed solution about it.

Three competing discourses for explaining inequalities (Carlisle, 2001) can be remembered using the mnemonics RED, SID and MUD.

Discourse level	Source of problem	Explanatory level	Causal mechanism	Solution level	Action
RED	Concentration of resources in higher socioeconomic (SE) groups	Social structure (SS)	Inequitable social distribution of resources	Redistribute resources downwards	Socioeconomic policy
SID	Social polarisation of SE groups	Interaction between individual and SS	Relative inequality and social stress in disadvantaged groups	Reduce gap and increase social integration	Community
MUD	Lower SE groups	Individual experience and action	Narrow resource margins	Help poor people develop their coping strategies	Individual

Table 4.1: Mnemonics for explaining inequalities

- **Red**istribution;
- **S**ocial **I**ntegrationist;
- **M**oral **U**nderclass.

Those who adhere to the RED discourse see the issue as one where resources are not scarce; rather, it is an issue of politics and policy which results in an unequal distribution of wealth and income. The problem is that the material resources for a healthy life are concentrated in the hands of those at the top of the social structure. It is the social structure (e.g. class structures, gender and ethnic structures) which is the root cause of this wealth and income inequality. The reason why people at the bottom are in poorer health is because of this inequity of distribution of resources. The answer is, by state intervention and social policies, to redistribute resources and challenge social structures (such as increasing social mobility so that one does not get stuck at the bottom) so that those at the bottom get a fairer share and increase their life chances. The discourse would emphasise words such as 'social structure'.

Those who adhere to the SID approach would see the issue of the relative positioning of socio-economic groups one to another rather than issues of resources being owned by the wealthy. Inequalities arise and are caused because social groups see and feel these relative differences between them. So the answer is to reduce the gap (maybe by creating employment opportunities and welfare benefits, tax credits at the bottom and caps in high earnings at the top). Community development work would be needed to address the perceptions of gaps and bring people together. The discourse may emphasise words such as 'community engagement'.

Those who adhere to the MUD discourse see the issue as a problem with the lower socioeconomic groups themselves. They are in poor health because of their own experiences, actions, attitudes and behaviours. This results in them not having much left over (if anything) after paying for basics. The solution is focusing at the individual level to provide education so that they choose healthier foods and activities, and stop smoking, taking drugs and drinking to excess. The discourse would emphasise words such as 'personal responsibility'.

This is, of course, a simplification of what actually happens.

Activity 4.3 — *Critical thinking*

Consider the Coalition government's ideas of the 'Big Society' and the 'Responsibility Deal'. Which, if any, of RED, SID or MUD applies to these ways of thinking?

An outline answer to this activity is given at the end of the chapter.

The existence of competing discourses explaining inequalities in health does not mean that each is equally valid. Just as in the 'debate' over anthropogenic climate change, the existence of contrary voices does not mean that the evidence is balanced or valid.

No doubt individuals make 'silly' choices, although the 'silliness' of, for example, smoking is, in the end, a value position. However, as Morrall argues:

the most mendacious game is that of instructing individuals to become more healthy when a major contributor to illness is social inequality. People need to stop smoking, avoid harmful food and exercise more habitually. But society also needs to reform its structures and surrounding by providing better housing, meaningful employment, adequate wages, improved working conditions, efficient transport systems and an unpolluted environment.
(Morrall, 2001, p. 195)

In the arena of population well-being and health there are very different ways of understanding what is and should be healthy. This will become much clearer as you study ideas that underpin public health theory and practice.

Historic (UK) publications

These important reports have outlined the policy discussions and answers to inequalities over the past few decades. They show the thinking behind what governments and individuals should do.

Inequalities in Health (*The Black Report*) (Townsend, 1988)

The main conclusion from this report was that the main explanation for inequalities was *material deprivation*. The social environment, which includes things like family size, unemployment, housing and income, impacts negatively on health. The mechanisms involved may include release of stress hormones as a result of material living conditions and, of course, lack of resources to buy low-fat, low-sugar, low-cholesterol nutritious food.

The Acheson Report (1998)

This report concurred with the *Black Report* of a decade earlier. It also found that the gap between the top and bottom socioeconomic groups had widened.

The Wanless Report (2003)

This report emphasised *layers of influence* – a theory that combines lifestyle choices, behaviours and environmental explanations for inequalities.

The Marmot Review (2010)

In November 2008, Professor Sir Michael Marmot was asked by the Secretary of State for Health to chair an independent review to propose the most effective *evidence-based* strategies for reducing health inequalities in England from 2010. The strategy includes policies and interventions that address the *social determinants* of health inequalities.

The Review had four tasks:

1. Identify, for the health inequalities challenge facing England, the evidence most relevant to underpinning future policy and action.
2. Show how this evidence could be translated into practice.
3. Advise on possible objectives and measures, building on the experience of the current targets on infant mortality and life expectancy.
4. Publish a report of the review's work that will contribute to the development of a post-2010 health inequalities strategy.

In February 2010, the Marmot Review Team published *Fair Society, Healthy Lives*. The report and further detail can be found at **www.marmotreview.org**.

The executive summary argued:

> *People with higher socioeconomic position in society have a greater array of life chances and more opportunities to lead a flourishing life. They also have better health. The two are linked: the more favoured people are, socially and economically, the better their health. This link between social conditions and health is not a footnote to the 'real' concerns with health – health care and unhealthy behaviours – it should become the main focus. Consider one measure of social position: education. People with university degrees have better health and longer lives than those without. For people aged 30 and above, if everyone without a degree had their death rate reduced to that of people with degrees, there would be 202,000 fewer premature deaths each year. Surely this is a goal worth striving for.* (Marmot, 2010, p. 3)

Fair Society, Healthy Lives (Marmot, 2010): Key messages of the Review

1. Reducing health inequalities is a matter of fairness and social justice. In England, the many people who are currently dying prematurely each year as a result of health inequalities would otherwise have enjoyed, in total, between 1.3 and 2.5 million extra years of life.
2. There is a social gradient in health – the lower a person's social position, the worse his or her health. Action should focus on reducing the gradient in health.
3. Health inequalities result from social inequalities. Action on health inequalities requires action across all the social determinants of health.
4. Focusing solely on the most disadvantaged will not reduce health inequalities sufficiently. To reduce the steepness of the social gradient in health, actions must be universal, but with a scale and intensity that are proportionate to the level of disadvantage. We call this proportionate universalism.
5. Action taken to reduce health inequalities will benefit society in many ways. It will have economic benefits in reducing losses from illness associated with health inequalities.

These currently account for productivity losses, reduced tax revenue, higher welfare payments and increased treatment costs.

6. Economic growth is not the most important measure of our country's success. The fair distribution of health, well-being and sustainability are important social goals. Tackling social inequalities in health and tackling climate change must go together.

7. Reducing health inequalities will require action on six policy objectives:

   - Give every child the best start in life.
   - Enable all children, young people and adults to maximise their capabilities and have control over their lives.
   - Create fair employment and good work for all.
   - Ensure healthy standard of living for all.
   - Create and develop healthy and sustainable places and communities.
   - Strengthen the role and impact of ill health prevention.

8. Delivering these policy objectives will require action by central and local government, the NHS, the third and private sectors and community groups. National policies will not work without effective local delivery systems focused on health equity in all policies.

9. Effective local delivery requires effective participatory decision making at local level. This can only happen by empowering individuals and local communities.

Implications for nursing practice

Dahlgren and Whitehead (1991) outlined a model for the social determinants of health which was developed by the United Kingdom Public Health Association strategic interest group in 2006 (Barton and Grant, 2006). These are what have been called the *causes of the causes*: the social, environmental, economic conditions that heavily influence (hence determine) the health of individuals and populations. Barton and Grant's (2006) 'health map' builds on this idea.

The Commission on the Social Determinants of Health takes a *holistic* view of social determinants of health. It argues that the unequal distribution of power, resources, wealth income and services across the globe have a direct effect on the health of the poor and result in a social gradient in health within countries and between countries. In addition, inequities in health are not natural or inevitable; they are a result of economic, political and policy failures.

The Commission on the Social Determinants of Health also argues that *the global community can put this right but it will take urgent and sustained action, globally, nationally, and locally.*

Traditionally, society has looked to the health sector to deal with its concerns about health and disease. Unequal access to health services is one of the social determinants of health. However, the high burden of illness responsible for premature loss of life arises because of the conditions in which people are born, grow, live, work and age.

Therefore, action on the social determinants of health must involve the whole of government, civil society and local communities, business, global forums and international agencies. The ministers of health and national departments of health are also critical to global change. The UK Department of Health and the UK nursing profession (in the form of the Royal College of Nursing, the NMC and nurses' participation in various public health bodies) could champion the social determinants of health approach.

The social determinants of health approach thus challenges the notion that health is the sole domain of the NHS and brings it squarely into the arena of local government and other agencies. For example, the *Foresight Report* (Aylott et al., 2008) argues that obesity cannot be addressed by the NHS alone. The report makes clear that the overwhelming scientific consensus is that 'modern life' is a major driver of obesity. Roberts and Edwards (2010) specifically suggest fossil fuel use, and especially the car, is also implicated in the rise of obesity in populations. Very importantly, for the health promotion role of the nurse, the report concludes that individual responsibility is important but insufficient to tackle obesity on its own. Nurses who thus focus only on changing individual behaviour have missed the point.

Davidson (2015) clearly outlines this argument, and refers to the *common sense or conventional model* of health and disease. This focuses on individual behaviour change based on a host–agent model whereby we are the 'host' and threats that might assault us are 'agents'. This model uses risk factor analysis and epidemiological data to explicate the causes and variations in frequency of disease and illness. It also relies too much on rational choice theory to underpin behaviour changes. For Davidson, both adopting healthy lifestyles and behaviour change theories are only marginally effective on health outcomes. Far more pertinent to our health is our social position and the *social patterning of behaviour.* Davidson refers to the work of Andree Demers to illustrate that point (see Activity 4.4).

It could be argued, therefore, that the NHS has a relatively minor role in addressing health inequalities and the social determinants of health. Nurses from this perspective thus are currently focused more on disease and illness rather than addressing the foundations for health. There is a need for nursing to understand the social and ecological determinants of health to rethink their health promotion role (Goodman, 2015). The NMC standards seem to recognise this in its statements on requirements for content of courses and in the generic domains. So what may nurses do to address these issues?

The NMC's generic standard for competence states:

> *All nurses must . . . promote health and wellbeing. All nurses must also understand how behaviour, culture, socioeconomic and other factors, in the care environment and its location, can affect health, illness, health outcomes and public health priorities and take this into account in planning and delivering care.*
>
> *. . . all nurses must also understand how behaviour, culture, socioeconomic and other factors, in the care environment and its location, can affect health, illness, health outcomes and public health priorities and take this into account in planning and delivering care.*
> (NMC, 2010, pp. 17, 26, 35, 44)

The Royal College of Nursing (2003, p. 3) definition of practice includes management, teaching, policy and knowledge development, in addition to direct patient care. Therefore, when you are observing, discussing and reading about, for example, clinical leadership, you are practising nursing. When you critique public health approaches, when you address issues such as homelessness or domestic violence, you are practising nursing. This is based on an understanding that nursing practice – in primary care as well as in hospitals – has to address illness and disease all the way through to health and well-being.

This is implicitly recognised in the NMC standards when the domain above states you must *understand*. The social sciences assist in this understanding. However, understanding without action may be an abrogation of our moral responsibility as healthcare professionals to address the very real health issues people face both in the UK and internationally.

So, for clarity, the frame of reference here is that healthy lives depend on a healthy socioeconomic and physical environment, as outlined in the social determinants of health approach, and as is explicit in Roper et al.'s (2000) model. Nursing cannot be immune from issues arising from social structure. It is not enough to learn how the body works and what to do when it goes wrong. Nurses have for a long time been pioneers for social action, acting on behalf of the poor, weak and vulnerable. Nightingale's focus on the patient and the immediate environment linked the two. Nursing theory and practice may need to develop further a critical edge, applying a psychosociological imagination that adds to the concepts of person, health, nursing and environment to embrace explicitly a sociopolitical dimension to the relationship between environment and health (Goodman, 2015).

A review of major nursing theorists (for example, Nightingale, Henderson, Hall, Watson) suggests an understanding of the link between social structure, individual psychology and environmental effects on health.

The following theorists come close to putting the links together. Martha Rogers' *science of unitary beings* suggests the existence of *energy fields* manifest in unitary human beings and environment. Callista Roy's (1980) *adaptation model* emphasises a biopsychosocial adaptive system within *an environment*. Madeleine Leininger's (1995) *transcultural nursing* (while focusing on care as the essence and distinctive feature of nursing which may improve human conditions) makes a step towards making the link between social structure and health. Rosemarie Parse's notion of *indivisible being and environment* suggests nurses assist with clients in interaction with environment while *co-creating health*.

A model of nursing that gets closer to discussion of the psychosocial issues is that of Roper et al. (2000). Interestingly, Nancy Roper has suggested disappointment in the way the model has been used in the UK (Siviter, 2002). This was based on *the lack of the application* of five important factors to the activities of daily living, factors which make the model holistic, resulting in incomplete and flawed assessments based on the model. Alongside the biological factors are the psychological and sociocultural factors. The environmental factors, Roper believed, make hers the first truly 'green' model, as it recommends consideration of not only the impact of the environment on the activities of daily living, but also the impact of the individual's activities of daily living on the environment.

The final factor in the model is the politico-economic. This is the impact of government, politics and the economy. This would address issues such as funding, government policies and programmes, state of war or violent conflict, availability and access to benefits, political reforms and government targets, interest rates and availability of public and private-sector funding.

Roper's model could thus be used as a basis for nurses to address a more holistic, or critical, approach to nursing. However, even though the environmental and politico-economic factors are highlighted, Roper's disappointment with the lack of application begs the question as to why this is so. One reason may be the dominance of biomedical paradigms, NHS priorities and competence-based education. It may also be ideological. Davidson (2015) clearly makes the links between health and the politics of neoliberalism and globalisation. He argues that action on the social determinants of health is often framed within the ideology of free-market capitalism, which is critical of using state intervention in public health matters beyond providing health services and arguing for the adoption by individuals of healthy lifestyles and improving their choices.

Action by nurses on behalf of, for example, what Paul Collier (2007) identifies as the *bottom billion* (that is, the very poorest people in the world) will not take place unless the social nature of health and illness is comprehended and owned. Progressive, liberal and humanist philosophies of education need to balance purely practical and vocationalist tendencies of nursing if there is to be a moral imperative to act to alter the social conditions which frequently are the origins of disease and death. The major social condition is the unequal power–wealth dynamic (World Health Organization, 2008; Horton et al., 2014; Ottersen et al., 2014; Davidson, 2015). Nursing theory is in danger of being neglected, with any critique of the existing unjust order that may have been present being lost. Nursing theory will have to rediscover its own critical edge, assuming it ever had one, if it is to contribute solutions and galvanise action to the 'messy' problems of the world. The challenge here is to decide at what level the practice should take place: individual, organisational, national and/or international? Practice will also depend on what field of nursing one enters and what clinical setting.

Activity 4.4   *Reflection*

Are we independent, autonomous actors or social creatures?

Andree Demers, a Canadian researcher, suggested that the amount of alcohol drank by students depended on the situation. The critical variables involved were: the friends they were drinking with, how much those friends drank, when and where the drinking took place. *It is apparent that the individual cannot be conceptualized as an autonomous actor* (Demers et al., 2002).

What does this mean? To what degree are our actions socially structured rather than a result of free choice? See Chapter 11 in Davidson (2015).

As this activity is your own reflection there is no outline answer at the end of the chapter.

If health has social determinants and if nurses are interested in promoting health, then it follows that nurses ought to consider their response to factors that go beyond the individual and the biological. This accords with the whole theme of this book, in that a psychosocial understanding is crucial to a more holistic view of health, illness and disease. Understanding the factors is one step; taking action to address them is another. The nature of that action is up to individual nurses and nursing organisations.

Chapter summary

- There are global health inequities which result in varying burdens of disease and life expectancy.
- The global pattern of inequalities is repeated within the UK.
- There are various explanations given for this that range from individual choice to social structure.
- Various discourses are used to support these explanations.
- Nursing practice in the face of these issues may require responsive action.

Activities: brief outline answers

Activity 4.1 Research and evidence-based practice

Millennium Development Goals

1. End poverty and hunger.
2. Universal education.
3. Gender equality.
4. Child health.
5. Maternal health.
6. Combat HIV/AIDS.
7. Environmental sustainability.
8. Global partnership.

Activity 4.2 Critical thinking and team working

Considering the question: 'Do poverty and ill health arise from the failings of individuals or from failings of society?', you and your colleagues might come up with something along the following lines:

On the one hand, not actively seeking work and drawing benefits is a moral failing, and shows that one is not trying hard enough, especially when there are plenty of jobs to be had. Immigrants get work so why can't UK nationals? Therefore being poor results from fecklessness.

On the other hand, when joblessness reaches three million and many new 'jobs' are actually temporary and part-time as well as being very low paid, combined with whole industries declining, then the individual gets caught up in larger social forces at play.

Activity 4.3 Critical thinking

The RED discourse is not really applicable in that the solution to 'Broken Britain' is not wealth redistribution. The answer lies in civil society, charities and volunteers, people 'doing it for themselves'. The 'Responsibility Deal' also is an individualist approach and thus borrows from the MUD discourse as it suggests that following education, the individual should take responsibility for health choices.

Further reading

Davidson, A (2015) *Social Determinants of Health: A Comparative Approach.* Oxford: Oxford University Press.

Provides a useful introduction to the subject.

Tschudin, V and Davis, A (2008) *The Globalisation of Nursing.* Oxford: Radcliffe.

An overview of the challenges facing the nursing profession in the twenty-first century.

Useful websites

www.gapminder.org

You may find Hans Rosling's Gapminder site a very good resource for gathering information on the state of the world's health. See, for example, the section entitled, 'Is child mortality falling?'

http://www.bbc.co.uk/programmes/b00v6lkp

Radio 4's *Analysis* (2010): *The Spirit Level: The Theory of Everything?* is available as a podcast.

http://www.bbc.co.uk/programmes/b01mw15s

Radio 4's *Analysis* (2012): *Social Epidemiology* is also available as a podcast.

www.equalitytrust.org.uk

Visit the Equality Trust for a wealth of information and indicators.

www.who.int/social_determinants/en

For World Health Organization social determinants of health.

http://www.apho.org.uk/default.aspx?RID=49802

Community health profiles indicate areas of relative social deprivation and health outcomes.

Chapter 5
Decision making

Chapter aims

After reading this chapter, you will be able to:

- understand why it is important to have the right information before making decisions;
- distinguish between 'good' and 'bad' science, and discuss the merits of basing your decisions on scientific knowledge;
- understand how the sociological and psychological context might contribute to decision making;
- explain the relationship between psychology, sociology and making decisions about patient care.

Introduction

Nurses are required to undertake practice and make decisions underpinned by the best available evidence. However, there are social issues around what is accepted as evidence, how that evidence gets used and who accepts what is evidence. Contemporary arguments (Goldacre, 2008; Singh and Ernst, 2008) exist around the use of complementary and alternative medicines (CAMs), around science as the only arbiter for knowledge creation upon which we base our evidence, and around the political nature of scientific evidence use (Pielke, 2010). To illustrate these points we will briefly explore how science 'works'. International drug policy will be used as an example of how evidence gets used and affected by policy decisions and value positions taken by those who make policy. We will also look at the relationship with national and international guidelines.

Not only is the evidence affected by external value positions and social influences, it is also affected by psychological issues – the 'cognitive structures' in our head or the way we think. We therefore need to explore how we go about making decisions and our errors in thinking, i.e. 'heuristics' and the mental 'short cuts' that cognitive science demonstrates are part and parcel of human thinking.

People also make decisions about their health status and behaviours. What do we think we know about this? We will briefly review some theories of rational action as applied to health behaviours.

Errors in thinking

Why do doctors make mistakes? Jerome Groopman (2008), Professor of Medicine at Harvard Medical School, USA, argues that most medical errors are not technical, but cognitive – in other words, errors of thinking. His book, *How Doctors Think*, identifies several forms of cognitive bias commonly encountered in the medical profession and makes practical suggestions for patients to help their doctor avoid such mistakes.

If doctors make mistakes based on errors in thinking, then so can nurses. However, this is not about having the correct knowledge base; this is about how our brains actually work in applying knowledge.

For example, a common error in thinking is 'confirmation bias'; that is, our tendency to see and accept evidence that supports our theory and ignore evidence that contradicts it. You have already encountered 'attribution error' (p. 61) as another example.

Daniel Kahneman in *Thinking, Fast and Slow* (2011) suggests that we have two modes of thought:

1. system 1: fast, automatic, frequent, emotional, stereotypic, subconscious, instinctive;
2. system 2: slow, effortful, infrequent, logical, calculating, conscious, more deliberative.

Both systems are prone to cognitive errors, a conclusion Kahneman reaches following several decades of academic research. He suggests that we place too much confidence in human judgement, and one reason we do so is because we use heuristics or mental short cuts. We will return to this idea later in this chapter.

Science and knowledge

What is science? How do we decide between different knowledge claims to truth? This is crucial for what we count as true, for what we count as our knowledge then becomes our evidence. Science provides one form of evidence. Experience provides another.

The scientific method is accepted by many, but not all, as the best route to truth and knowledge that we have. It is not perfect, as science is indeed open to social influences and interests that shape what gets investigated, how it gets investigated and how that knowledge is accepted or used. Oreskes and Conway (2010) in their book *Merchants of Doubt* describe how science can be distorted or used to deny certain positions. They suggest that the US scientific community has a strong record of research on public health, environmental science and other issues affecting the quality of life. Scientists have been producing studies on the dangers of DDT, tobacco smoke, acid rain and global warming over many years. Yet it remains the case that a powerful subset of scientists leads the world in strong denial of these dangers. The suggestion is that some of this science is distorted to support corporate interests. That being said, that is a not a critique of the scientific method per se, just the uses that science gets put to.

It is important thus to distinguish between how science is practised and reported, which undoubtedly has sociopolitical influences; see the discussion on drugs policy below, and the truth claims of science itself.

Sociologists have been debating scientific knowledge, with some arguing for the social construction of science. The strong, or postmodern, version of this insists that there is no such thing as objective reality out there waiting to be discovered, and existing independently of human understanding. In this sense there is no empirical world of physical objects. All reality is mediated through human consciousness, how individuals perceive what they are seeing and feeling, and thus reality becomes social in that to get an agreement on what exists, humans get together to construct what it is they think they are experiencing.

For the social constructionist the social world feels real because we decide it is real. Postmodernists take social construction one step further. Science is not real; it has no more validity than any form of knowledge. Everything in the social and natural world is only a product of the human mind. Thus, there can never be any external facts or universal laws because human cultures construct their natural and social worlds so differently. All systems of belief, e.g. science and religion, are merely human constructions and one cannot take primacy over another. If they do so it is because of the exercise of power, which enables certain social groups to impose their system of belief on others.

Concept summary: Empiricism

'Empiricalitis' implies a criticism of evidence-based practice, or rather the attitude towards it that elevates it above all other bases for knowledge. The 'evidence base' is rooted in a particular form of science, i.e. 'empiricism', that is itself only one way of understanding the world.

The core idea of empiricism is that only, or primarily, human sensory experience, what we see with our eyes, for example, is the basis for knowledge. It thus emphasises the role of experience and evidence in the formation of ideas and knowledge. Scientific experimentation is a method used to generate knowledge, and thus if science can't measure it, it cannot be real. Any theory must be tested in the 'real' world of sensory experience.

The critique is not that this approach by itself is wrong but that too much importance is placed upon it at the expense of theory or reason, thereby overlooking the role of the social context and social influences on human behaviour. Other forms of knowledge – intuition, argument, inspiration, artistry or custom – are overlooked or ridiculed, leading to an over-reliance on this form of science (Morrall, 2009).

In the natural sciences such as physics and biology empiricism works well up to a point; at the quantum level it does not. In the social sciences, however, human behaviour is not so open to measurements and prediction in the same manner.

Objections to science often rest upon an assumption that science deals in certainties. However, science is not merely empirical, delivering certain truths drawn from experimentation; it is always tentative and also draws upon theory and reasoning. Physicists can be divided into two 'camps': those carrying out experiments such as those at the Large Hadron Collider, and those engaged in theoretical, mathematically based work, such as that of Peter Higgs, who theorised back in the 1960s about the existence of what has been called the 'God' particle, known as the Higgs boson.

Nurses may be ambivalent about science (MacKay, 2010; Rolfe, 2010) in that traditional scientific methods are accepted on the one hand as the only path to truth (empiricalism), while being rejected on the other in the embrace of CAMs. There is ongoing debate in the literature around what counts as evidence and the relative strengths of quantitative statistical methods using randomised controlled trials (RCTs) and qualitative methods using interviews and patient stories. There is a hierarchy of evidence (Guyatt et al., 2008) which places the RCT as the gold standard at the top. Such things as 'opinions of experts' and 'patient anecdote' come below this. The debate is now less polarised than it used to be, with both methodologies coming together in some research projects.

Evidence for nurses

What counts as evidence for nurses? Of course, scientific knowledge counts, but so also do clinical experience, expert opinion, personal experience, intuition, patients' stories, custom, practice and ritual.

There may be something in the argument that suggests that knowledge arises out of social processes, from events (history) and from the influence of powerful groups who have influence over what gets accepted as true.

Consider situations in which nurses may find themselves. It is not the case that clinical nurses sit around poring over research papers before making decisions about what is in the best interest of patients. Most clinical practice consists of practical activity and discussion with colleagues and patients. This is a social process. It is not science. However, this social process 'produces' knowledge that the staff take as useful (or not) as the case may be. You may think of certain people – senior nurses, medics – in that social group who are listened to more than others and in doing so this helps to create 'knowledge'. The 'apprenticeship' system of 'see one, copy one, do one' passes on knowledge in this social way. Nurse 'training' produced its own knowledge in this way and in many ways still does.

This then makes using 'best available evidence' a critical activity because we have to check the knowledge we are using and ask ourselves upon what basis do we accept it? However, when it comes to choosing between certain therapies, we often rely on the products of scientific enquiry. Who now would choose leeches instead of drugs? Who would now administer water instead of drugs? Well, homeopaths, and some nurses who accept this therapy, may do so, but they do so confusing the specific effect of the potion based on the theory that water has a memory and that this memory of 'like cures like' is the specific effect with the net effect which includes placebos.

Randomised controlled trials and placebos

RCTs and placebos provide an example of confusing explanations for effectiveness.

Let us think about the effects of any drug or other intervention. The overall effect that a person experiences from a drug is called the 'net effect'. This is because there is a 'specific effect' which arises directly from the drug and there is also a 'context effect'. This context effect also includes placebo effects. So the net effect is context (and placebo) effect + specific effect.

So, when evaluating the usefulness of a drug or intervention we have to establish whether the measurable net effect (e.g. reduction in pain) resulting from a drug or a homeopathic remedy is either a specific effect of the drug itself and/or a multifactorial context net effect.

An RCT will measure the net effect but will be unable to distinguish between specific and context effects. So we have to be clear about the difference between these types of effect. To try to get around this, RCTs have to be sufficiently large to account for the many context effects involved. They then need to be repeated many times before a tentative conclusion can be reached.

Homeopathy, like medicine, claims specific effects – dilute solutions of 'like cures like' – but also context effects, i.e. the practitioner relationship and a holistic approach. It may well be that it is the context effect of homeopathic practice that accounts for the majority, if not all, of homeopathic healing. Context is a complex concept, but it may involve the physical environment of the clinic or hospital, the personality and demeanour of the practitioner, and the 'meanings response' held by patients – the meanings patients attach to things (Moerman, 2003). In a 1984 paper, Ulrich suggested that patients recover quicker following gall bladder surgery in a decent ward environment. This may be an example of a context effect. That is to say, it was not the ward itself but the totality of the ward, patient expectations, their meanings and how they felt.

RCTs may fail to consider the context effect of treatments, arguing that the net effect of interventions, that which is measured by an RCT, fails to pick up on the difficult-to-measure context effects which include placebo. Thus, positive trial results could include the specific effect of the drug plus the context and placebo effects, but because the latter are not measured the net effect is equated wrongly with the specific effect of the drug. In other words, RCTs may overplay the direct specific effects drugs have and downplay the effects that the context has. So drugs may not work in the way we think they do.

One theory for why a context effect may work is Porges' polyvagal theory and the ventral–vagal complex . The autonomic nervous system reacts to stimuli with the well-known 'flight or fight' response, but also with the ventral–vagal complex response, which triggers the nurturing system, i.e. the safety and contentment response rather than our stress response. A trigger could even be facial expressions and the sense of empathy and validation practitioners give to patients.

If nurses engage in any therapy, be it traditional medicine or CAMs, we need to be mindful of the knowledge that underpins it. However, realising that both scientific medicine and CAMs have their critiques should not lead to paralysis of action. We know enough about what works to begin the healing work of nursing. This should always be done with a critical eye on knowledge and truth claims and a realisation that not all truth claims are equal. This also applies to national policies and guidelines that may be open to various biases and influences.

Activity 5.1   *Research and evidence-based practice*

When next in clinical practice, identify any nursing intervention and then try to uncover what evidence is actually being used for it. Try to identify if the evidence comes from scientific trials or whether it is custom, or experience.

(For example, if you see that several patients are taking antidepressants, refer to the clinical evidence for the effectiveness of the medication and compare with what is actually happening.)

As this activity is based on your own experience and observations, there is no outline answer at the end of the chapter.

Learning nursing practice will involve you in studies based on the sciences and the scientific method. Often this will be understated as you learn the physiology of kidney function or the treatments for depression. Sometimes this will be explicit as you study evidence-based practice and learn about clinical trials or qualitative research. Alongside this you will read nursing theory that talks about the artistry of nursing practice, or intuition-based practice. You will come across arguments about how we know what we know about human life, health, disease and treatment/ therapies.

There are differing philosophies about 'understanding' and 'knowledge' and how we acquire them, and this often leads to discussion about the very essence of 'truth' – whether we can find it, or even if it exists at all.

There are also 'fashions' in academia which often shape the terms of debate. Back in the 1960s and 1970s it was very fashionable to study Marxism in sociology. Nursing today embraces many fashions – you will see that some nursing research likes to use 'phenomenology' and argues that this is a way forward for nursing to gain knowledge about humanity. Other researchers discuss 'postmodernism', while others tend towards quantitative methods and the use of trials. For some nurses, it seems that there is no one 'truth'.

In addition to all of this, some nurses look towards 'alternative' or 'complementary' therapies. The list ranges from acupuncture, reiki and homeopathy to 'crystal healing'. Underpinning these approaches is often a mistrust of allopathic or 'conventional' medicine and the scientific method. This mistrust is based on the often-agreed identified failings of conventional medicine, but perhaps more seriously, it is based on a disagreement about truth and how we come to know it. The scientific method, which has been the bedrock of many advances in human knowledge, is sometimes seen as merely a dominant ideology.

Evidence-based drug policy

The outcome of many, often small, studies in topics are such that often the ramifications of taking the research at face value are not socially or politically important. Pielke (2010) describes the relationship between public policy and scientific research as problematic, in that it is not a linear model in which scientists come up with answers which are then put into practice by policy makers. Pielke was using climate science as an example.

Evidence comes in many forms, not just science, but it is also naive to assume that if we have the evidence we will use it. It is the case that evidence gets ignored, distorted and misrepresented, sometimes with enormous consequences. It is not the case that science gives us the answers and then we implement policy based on that science. Often ideology trumps science. An example in health is the issue of substance use and abuse. The first point is that this can be seen as a criminal justice issue dealt with through law and courts or as a public health and welfare issue dealt with by health policies, or, of course, it can be a mixture of both. The research evidence includes studies into harms caused by substances, efficacy and cost-effectiveness of interventions and treatment options, education and prevention programmes.

However, this research field is characterised by ideology and politics, which operate in the background of many discussions. There is what some refer to as the 'prohibition church' (Cohen, 2003) which has set the international policy agenda. On the other hand, there are those, e.g. Transform Drug Policy Alliance, who call for alternative policies. There are those who state they just wish to conduct certain biochemical analyses free from political interference, e.g. the Independent Scientific Committee on Drugs. We need to think about what research does not say as much as what it does say, how it says it, who says it and what assumptions they hold.

For example, a distinction needs to be drawn between research that shows a substance to be harmful and research into the policy around that substance. A policy option of prohibition does not logically follow on from demonstrating harm. If harm alone was a criterion for banning something, then there is a case to be made for banning the car. The fact that we do not ban cars or motor cycles illustrates the multifactorial and political nature of such decisions. It may be relatively easy to show that a substance harms the user, although the case of ecstasy below shows otherwise; however, whether prohibition is the correct approach needs very careful research, including criteria such as social harm and unintended consequences of prohibition. Drug policy research falls into the category of public health research for which evidence for efficacy of options is often lacking (Baggot, 2010).

International drug policy

The overarching framework on drug regulation is the various United Nations conventions, with the USA particularly historically influential in setting the prohibitionist tone. It is therefore useful to consider a view from the USA. McCoun and Reuter (2008) suggested that there are *implicit rules* which govern the nature of research in the USA when it comes to drugs. In other words, anyone engaged in researching drugs in the USA has to abide by certain 'unwritten rules' to ensure their work remains within acceptable policy limits. For example, they argue that one of the rules that guides research is: *Evidence that an illicit drug could have benefits may not be collected.* They go on to list eight 'rules' in total. If they are correct, then it is imperative that our critical faculties are brought to bear when assessing US drugs research. It also begs the question as to whether these assumptions travel elsewhere.

Activity 5.2   *Critical thinking*

If substance use research is open to sociopolitical influence, what other areas of research and evidence gathering may be open to interests, omissions, interpretations? Can you think of any nursing (or any other) research which, while not overtly political in nature, may be open to social influences and/or repudiation of 'normal' science?

An outline answer to this activity is given at the end of the chapter.

Research summary: Drug policy

The US National Institute on Drug Abuse (NIDA) produced a report on MDMA (ecstasy). The 'political' nature of the report has been criticised by organisations such as Drugscope. To judge a substance's effect (and gauge its harm) we have to account not merely for its pharmacological content (although for certain substances that is clearly enough – arsenic, for example); we have to account for the mind set that users bring to it and the setting in which it is taken. This gives us the model: *drug, set and setting* (Zinberg, 1984). Alcohol taken in the form of one pre-dinner sherry (drug) by a usually abstemious (mind set) vicar only when visiting friends (setting) is certainly a different experience from that of young students having just passed exams (mind set) out on the town at happy hour (setting). Perrone (2005) argued that these factors are overlooked by US policy makers in their response to club drugs.

The difference between Drugscope's description and that of NIDA is the lack of hyperbole about abuse and a greater acceptance of uncertainty. The political nature of research was exemplified by Dr George A. Ricaurte, one of ecstasy's most vocal opponents in the scientific community. He admitted in the journal *Science* that a major study he had conducted (in 2002) proving the drug was dangerous when used on primates was in fact severely flawed. The drug Ricaurte used on the primates was not MDMA. Compelling evidence MDMA could permanently hurt the human brain could no longer be trusted as true. This report would have informed the NIDA report. A psychiatrist, Julie Holland (2003), has argued for the therapeutic use of MDMA but, mindful of the political ramifications of her stance, she emphasised the non-recreational use of MDMA.

The NIDA report (2006) can be found at **www.drugabuse.gov/publications/research-reports/mdma-ecstasy-abuse**

Drugscope's (2009) comments on ecstasy can be found at **www.drugscope.org.uk/resources/drugsearch/drugsearchpages/ecstasy**

Dr Ricaurte's study can be found at **www.mdma.net/toxicity/ricaurte.html**

Dr Holland's position can be found at **www.mdma.net/psychotherapy/index.html**

Case study: The Advisory Council on the Misuse of Drugs and Independent Scientific Council on Drugs

In the UK, the Advisory Council on the Misuse of Drugs (ACMD) states it is an independent body advising the government. It was established under the Misuse of Drugs Act 1971.

It states that it makes recommendations to government on the control of dangerous or otherwise harmful drugs, including classification and scheduling under the Misuse of Drugs Act 1971 and its regulations. It considers any substance which is being or appears to be being misused and which is having or appears to be capable of having harmful effects sufficient to cause a social problem.

It also carries out indepth inquiries into aspects of drug use that are causing particular concern in the UK, with the aim of producing considered reports that will be helpful to policy makers and practitioners.

continued . . . . . . •

The ACMD classification system was criticised as unscientific and arbitrary. Its work has been seen to be overly secretive and too close to government. Drug Classification: Making a Hash of It? *(2006) is the title of a report authored by the UK House of Commons Science and Technology Committee. The report suggested that the current system of recreational drug classification in the UK was arbitrary and unscientific (House of Commons Science and Technology Committee, 2006) and suggested a more scientific measure of harm be used for classifying drugs. The report also strongly criticised the decision to place fresh 'magic mushrooms' in class A, the same category as cocaine and heroin.*

In 2007, Professor David Nutt (chair of the ACMD) and colleagues published 'Development of a rational scale to assess the harm of drugs of potential misuse' (Nutt et al., 2007a), arguing that the Misuse of Drugs Act 1971 *is* not fit for purpose *and that* the exclusion of alcohol and tobacco from the Misuse of Drugs Act is, from a scientific perspective, arbitrary *(Nutt et al., 2007b).*

In February 2009 the UK government was then accused by David Nutt of making a political decision with regard to drug classification in rejecting the scientific advice to downgrade ecstasy from a class A drug. The ACMD (2008) report on ecstasy, based on a 12-month study of 4,000 academic papers, concluded that it is nowhere near as dangerous as other class A drugs such as heroin and crack cocaine, and should be downgraded to class B. The advice was not followed (Travis, 2009). Jacqui Smith, then Home Secretary, was also widely criticised by the scientific community for bullying Professor David Nutt into apologising for his previous comments that, in the course of a normal year, more people died from falling off horses (equasy or equine addiction syndrome) than died from taking ecstasy (Kmietowicz, 2009).

In 2009 Nutt was sacked by the Home Secretary Alan Johnson, who said:

It is important that the government's messages on drugs are clear and as an advisor you do nothing to undermine public understanding of them. I cannot have public confusion between scientific advice and policy and have therefore lost confidence in your ability to advise me as Chair of the ACMD.
(Easton, 2009; Tran, 2009)

In response, Nutt has set up the Independent Scientific Committee on Drugs, in an attempt to be free from political interference.

Ecstasy remains a class A drug despite Nutt's call for reclassification and evidence regarding its harms. The debate over cannabis continues.

The current situation

Drugs policy continues to be under the authority of United Nations conventions, although countries are beginning to try different approaches within the prohibitionist framework. There are continuing calls for policy to be evidence-based, for example, the Vienna Declaration (2010) and in the *BMJ* (Wood, 2010). In 2014 the Home Office published a report on international comparisons of drugs laws and suggested that tough laws are not related to lower levels of use (Home Office, 2014). The report was seen as an evidence-based position that challenged orthodox thinking on current UK drug legislation. However, to date it has not affected the legalisation or decriminalisation of illicit drugs in the UK.

Arguments continue over drug policy. Gyngell (2009), for example, argues that the current (prohibitionist) policy has not been implemented fully, and that liberalisation has crept into the UK's response. In *The Phoney War on Drugs* she argues for abandoning the harm reduction approach, focusing on all illicit drugs, encouraging programmes aimed at abstinence and rehabilitation, and funding a tougher and better enforcement regime to reduce supply. This is in opposition to arguments put forward, for example, by the Transform Drug Policy Foundation, which argues for regulation and control rather than continuing with the 'war on drugs'.

Clinical decision making, heuristics and cognitive bias

Now that we have raised the idea that social issues affect what counts as evidence and how evidence is used, we need to consider our individual thinking and explore how that directs decisions. Thus, we need to consider how we go about making decisions and reflect not just on external factors that impinge on our decision making but the internal or 'cognitive' factors that are involved. Some factors that are involved in our decision making include:

- The realisation that professional practice is not certain or always predictable, that is to say, that dealing with patients involves complexity and uncertainty. We are not machines and we don't react like machines. Consider the fact that even with drug therapy there are individual responses that surprise us.
- There is now within the NHS an 'evidence-based' culture, which means that as far as possible all action should have some evidence to support it and for many people this means scientific evidence drawn from clinical trials if possible.
- Alongside scientific evidence professionals use intuition and professional expertise, which are both important, but cannot be relied on.

What follows is by no means exhaustive, but offers an introduction to the large study of decision making, reasoning and exercising clinical judgement based upon insights from behavioural and cognitive psychology, and especially the work of Daniel Kahneman. A key message is that, although we may think we are rational in our decision making and weigh up evidence and argument before we decide to do something, the evidence actually suggests we let emotion and unconscious errors in thinking – cognitive biases – guide our decisions.

One way of looking at how we make these decisions is this: nurses use scientific knowledge in a clinical encounter with a patient which should lead to a uniformly optimal decision – that is to say, the same scientific knowledge used by another nurse in the same situation should provide the same result. However, this is a flawed linear model which inadequately describes the decision-making process.

Cognitive research understands the limitations of human cognition and emphasises our tendency to take mental short cuts.

The social context of decision making in which nurses and medical practitioners operate is dynamic and complex, which means that professionals have to take often difficult decisions quickly and in changing circumstances. The range of clinical settings (primary care – acute care, mental health, learning disabilities services) and patient conditions is vast and not all of them have easy, straightforward answers. The evidence base for a decision may be weak, unknown or inaccessible. In this context it has been suggested that professionals engage in 'heuristic' thinking as a way of simplifying the decision-making process. The notion of heuristics is important as it suggests there is a tendency to take short cuts in thinking due to external pressures.

Nurses use knowledge from their clinical experience to deal with the uncertainties they face. However, this way of making decisions can result in over-confidence in their own knowledge base, 'being correct after the event' or with the benefit of hindsight. The reliance on clinical experience means that nurses use short cuts which introduce biases into decision making.

Activity 5.3   *Reflection*

Identify short cuts in your own thinking – an obvious example from everyday life is driving your car. To what extent do we all stick strictly to all the rules of the Highway Code and in addition what information do we use when driving along a normal trunk road? Any discussion with an advanced motoring instructor about what cues we ought to use when making driving decisions will probably reveal our own short cuts and lack of knowledge.

As this activity is based on your own experience and observations, there is no outline answer at the end of the chapter.

Cognitive biases

Fundamental attribution error, discussed in Chapter 3, is one form of 'cognitive bias'. Other examples of cognitive biases are discussed in the following sections.

Dunning-Kruger effect

There is incompetence in the methods used to become successful at activities. This incompetence leads not just to failure but to misunderstanding the reasons for that failure. The incompetence works in these two ways and does not allow understanding of the real reasons for failure. It leads to false thinking that 'all is well', or 'it is someone else's fault'.

So, the inability to analyse a research paper accurately leads to not realising that an inaccurate understanding is created. A study is then critiqued on false grounds. For example, a small-scale qualitative research study (e.g. ten patients interviewed about their experiences of a diagnosis of cancer) is criticised for not producing results that can be generalised to the wider population.

The writers making this statement do not realise that this sort of study cannot and does not set out to generalise from only ten patients. Effectively, what the writers are doing here is the equivalent of criticising a lemon for not being a pear, but they do not realise it. That is the first incompetence. If this judgement was based on poor study techniques or an inability to understand research ideas and this inability is not realised, i.e. the students think they can understand the ideas quite well, then this is the second incompetence. The students will then blame failure not on their own inabilities but on, for example, poor teaching.

An example of the Dunning-Kruger effect occurs if a senior believes junior colleagues to be incompetent because they do not quickly come up with the answers to particular questions about patient care. The real reason for the junior staff members' behaviour may, in fact, be incompetence by the senior in the methods of asking for the answers to questions (for example, by being brusque, aggressive or intimidating). The senior's inability to see his or her own incompetence in asking patient care questions will prevent that person from seeing where the true error lies.

Base-rate neglect bias

This means forgetting the underlying base rate of disease or illness when diagnosing or treating. The base rate is the true number of patients in a population who have a disease or characteristic.

This list is not exhaustive, but it illustrates that our thinking processes are open to many different forms of error and bias. In developing critical thought we need to be able to understand that our thinking may not be as rational and evidence-based as we think it is, and then we need to begin to develop ways of thinking through which we challenge ourselves to clarify our errors. However, Kahneman admits that even awareness of these errors in our thinking does not necessarily stop us from falling into the trap. Knowledge alone is not enough.

Three common heuristics (short cuts in thinking)

Availability

This is a cognitive heuristic in which a decision maker relies upon knowledge that is readily available rather than examining other alternatives or procedures.

There are situations in which people assess the probability of an event by the ease with which instances or occurrences can be brought to mind. For example, one may assess the risk of heart attack among middle-aged people by recalling such occurrences among one's acquaintances or the statistical knowledge of heart attacks in that age group.

Availability is a useful clue for assessing frequency or probability. The available cue of central crushing chest pain in a middle-aged male smoker is useful in guiding assessment because probability directs us that way.

Representativeness

Many of the probabilistic questions with which people are concerned belong to one of the following types: What is the probability that object A belongs to class B? What is the probability that event A originates from process B? What is the probability that process B will generate event A? In answering such questions, people typically rely on the representativeness heuristic, in which probabilities are evaluated by the degree to which A is representative of B, that is, by the degree to which A resembles B. For example, when A is highly representative of B, the probability that A originates from B is judged to be high. On the other hand, if A is not similar to B, the probability that A originates from B is judged to be low.

What is the probability that unconsciousness (object A) originates from hypoglycaemia (process B), if the nature of the unconsciousness is representative of similar events that result from hypoglycaemia (for example, is accompanied by a low blood glucose reading)?

What is the probability that hearing voices (object A) originates from schizophrenia (process B) if the nature of those voices is representative of similar episodes that result from schizophrenia (for example, is accompanied by delusions)?

How may representativeness of this nature mislead?

Anchoring or focalism

This describes the common human tendency to rely too heavily, or 'anchor', on one trait or piece of information when making decisions. During normal decision making, individuals anchor, or overly rely, on specific information or a specific value and then adjust to that value to account for other elements of the circumstance. Usually, once the anchor is set, there is a bias towards that value.

Take, for example, a person looking to buy a used car – the person may focus excessively on the milometer reading and model year of the car, and use those criteria as a basis for evaluating the value of the car, rather than considering how well the engine or the gearbox is maintained.

Scenario

An elderly woman has fallen and is unable to get up from the floor. There is obvious shortening and rotation of her leg, indicating a hip fracture. This may then provide the 'anchor' to guide subsequent treatment options at the expense of assessing for predisposing factors for the fall (such as a transient ischaemic attack).

Experiments in cognitive science and social psychology have revealed a wide variety of biases in areas such as statistical reasoning, social attribution and memory. These biases are common to all human beings, and some have been demonstrated to hold across very different cultures.

If short cuts and biases in ways of thinking can occur, then this may also apply to the sources of evidence we use for decision making.

Research summary: Stages in the reasoning process

There are various descriptions of how we go about reasoning. Some descriptions are linear, so we need to reflect on how well they match actual reality.

Elstein et al. (1978) Medical Problem Solving: An Analysis of Clinical Reasoning

1. Cue acquisition – this patient has chest pain, radiating to neck and arm.
2. Hypothesis generation – this event is cardiac in origin.
3. Cue interpretation – the nature of the pain looks like that associated with a myocardial infarction (MI).
4. Hypothesis evaluation – if this is an MI, the electrocardiogram (ECG) should show ST elevation, which supports or throws doubt on my hypothesis.

Carnevali (1984) Diagnostic Reasoning in Nursing

1. Exposure to pre-encounter data. The statistics and knowledge around ischaemic heart disease: patients with MI present with particular clinical signs and symptoms, usually within a specific age range and often have predisposing risk factors. This is pre-existing knowledge of cardiac conditions that the practitioner has.
2. Entry to the data field and shaping the direction of data gathering. This patient is 54 years old, overweight and a smoker (three aspects of the 'data field'). He is complaining of chest pain. Therefore, data should be gathered around vital signs, lab tests, ECGs, lifestyle cues and description of pain.
3. Coalescing of cues into data clusters. The physiological data are put together. The social and family history is put together.
4. Hypothesis – this patient has an MI.
5. Hypothesis search of the data field. Are there any more data that can be gathered which will confirm or deny the hypothesis? Thinking that this is an MI will lead one to look for certain information.
6. Testing hypothesis data for fit. Does the hypothesis fit the data clusters?
7. Diagnosis – MI.

How do Elstein et al.'s and Carnevali's outlines of decision making describe what actually happens? Are these 'normative' theories (that is, a theory about how decisions *should* be made) as opposed to 'descriptive' theories (that is, how decisions are actually made)?

| Activity 5.4 | *Decision making* |

Think of a patient/client scenario you have encountered recently which necessitated your making a clinical decision. What steps did you take to reach your decision? Provide a rationale. Consider how much emphasis you attribute to each piece of clinical information and articulate your reasons.

How would you improve your own decision-making process?

An outline answer to this activity is given at the end of the chapter.

The cognitive continuum (intuition–analysis)

Thinking is affected by our thinking processes and by external factors. We may think intuitively ('on our feet', which then may let in cognitive bias and heuristics) or we may think analytically, weighing up all the science and evidence before acting. The cognitive continuum (Hamm, 1988), revised for nursing by Standing (2008), is a model to explain or perhaps predict what sort of thinking we will engage in based on the situation in which we find ourselves. The argument here is that the major determinant of whether a practitioner uses intuitive or analytical thinking is the position of the decision task on a continuum. This depends on: (1) the structure of the task; (2) number of information cues; and (3) the time available to make judgements (Figure 5.1).

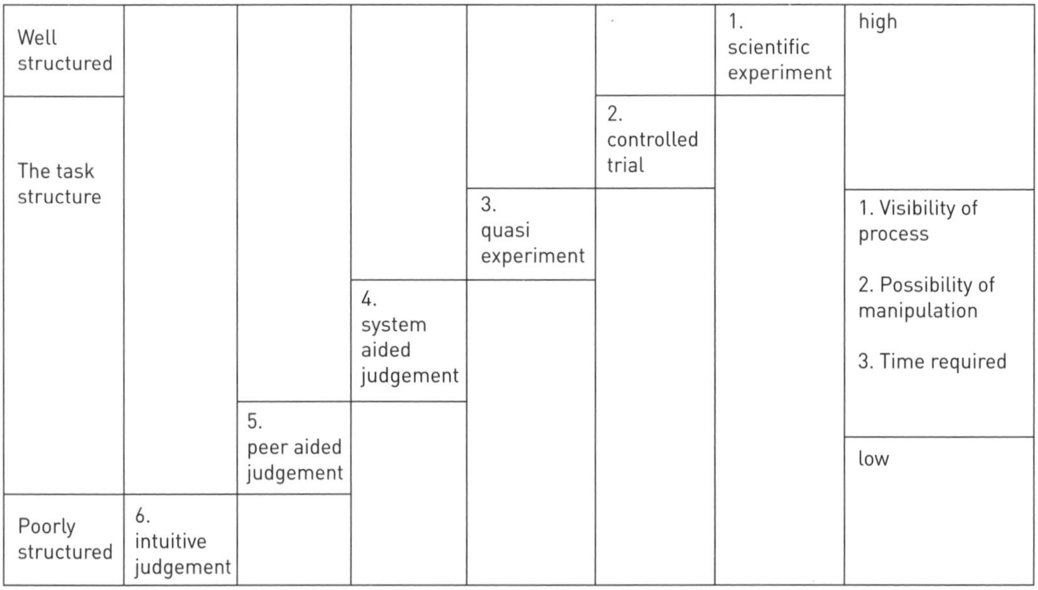

Well structured						1. scientific experiment	high
The task structure					2. controlled trial		
				3. quasi experiment			1. Visibility of process
			4. system aided judgement				2. Possibility of manipulation
							3. Time required
		5. peer aided judgement					low
Poorly structured	6. intuitive judgement						

Figure 5.1: The cognitive continuum (based on the ideas of Hamm, 1988)

It is suggested that most healthcare interventions fall in the middle of the continuum, so a systems-aided judgement is the most appropriate form of cognition. Thus, a poorly structured task with many information cues and very little time suggests intuition as the appropriate/usual mode of cognition.

Is there a possibility, therefore, that certain clinical scenarios push practitioners towards intuitive judgements instead of towards a more analytical approach?

> ## Scenario A: A poorly structured task
>
> *A patient who is drunk complains of pain. Assessing, examining, diagnosing and treating abdominal pain, you are asked to perform multiple functions which may not have clear-cut dimensions to them.*
>
> *There are many information cues: the look of the patient, the patient's descriptions of pain, the clinical parameters, the patient's attitude and demeanour, investigations results.*
>
> *There is time for a 10-minute consultation before the next patient turns up. You have a waiting room of anxious, increasingly resentful patients.*

> ## Scenario B: A highly structured task
>
> *You have been tasked (with the mother's consent) with the administration of an MMR vaccination.*
>
> *The only information cue is the age of the patient and the recorded need for MMR. There is no other presenting illness or injury.*
>
> *The vaccinations are not due until next week. You have plenty of time to decide if this is the right course of action.*

Decision making and health beliefs

The decisions we make about health are influenced by many factors, social, political, cultural and individual beliefs. Pescosolido (2000) outlines four models of health and illness behaviour that try to answer the question about how we come to recognise and adapt to health problems and issues.

The following four models can be found on the Open University's 'Open learn': Issues in Complementary and Alternative Medicine (**http://www.open.edu/openlearn/health-sports-psychology/health/health-studies/issues-complementary-and-alternative-medicine/content-section-1.4**).

The socio-behavioural model (SBM)

The SBM details three basic categories: need, predisposing characteristics and enabling factors. *Need for care* must be established, and this depends on the nature of the illness and its severity (for example, the 'hurt', 'worry', 'bother' or 'pain' that it causes). The SBM considers how people perceive this need and how symptoms are experienced. *Predisposing characteristics* include gender, ethnicity, education and beliefs: that is, the social and cultural factors which shape an individual's tendency to seek care. *Enabling characteristics* recognise that individuals need to act on a desire to receive care, and include the means and knowledge to get treatment (having a source of care, travel time and financial ability, as well as the geographical availability of doctors and clinics). A nurse working with a patient might have to consider whether the 'need for care' has in fact been established, especially in terms of issues such as smoking cessation. If smoking is not currently causing any health issues it might be that a 'need for care' is dismissed by the individual.

The health belief model (HBM)

Whereas the SBM focuses on the influence of the system and issues of access, the HBM examines the meaning of 'predisposing' characteristics and analyses how an individual's specific health beliefs (for example, about the severity of symptoms) and preferences (for example, the perceived benefits of treatment), as well as experiences (with healthcare problems and providers and the patient's knowledge), affect decisions to seek care and adopt health behaviours. For people gaining weight leading to obesity in the future, their decisions may be based on certain core beliefs about how and why weight gain occurs. Their intake of high-sugar-content carbonated drinks may not feature in their personal assessments of weight gain. Instead it may be put down to 'hormones'.

The theory of reasoned action (TRA)

The TRA concerns *expectancy*: individuals rate how current and alternative actions can reduce their health problems. Like the HBM, this theory focuses on motivations, the individual's assessment of risk and the desire to avoid negative outcomes. Individuals evaluate whether or not to engage in healthy (for example, taking exercise) or risky (for example, smoking) behaviours and whether to seek preventive as well as curative medical services.

The theory of planned behaviour (TPB)

The TPB evolved from the TRA, but differs by recognising that individuals do not necessarily have control over their behaviour. The amount of behavioural control – or self-efficacy – that individuals perceive they have is an important element in this model. Also, 'cues' or 'habits' become an important part of the decisions individuals make to engage in health and illness behaviours (adapted from Pescosolido, 2000, pp. 176–177).

The above approach however has been criticised for over-emphasising rational action and downplaying other cultural, political, cognitive and personal factors that impact on our decision making about our health. They may have some usefulness as guidance and health professionals might consider their use in helping people to make better decisions. 'Rational choice' as a mechanism may not actually be what happens in people's lives. The discussion of cognitive biases illustrates that rationality and conscious decision making are not necessarily an accurate picture of our thinking. See Chapter 11 in Davidson (2015) for a critique.

Activity 5.5   *Critical thinking*

Using the cognitive continuum, what can you say about the possibility and characteristic of the cognitive mode that each scenario above suggests? (That is to say, will the use of intuition or analysis come to the fore?) What is the implication of your answer for clinical practice?

An outline answer to this activity is given at the end of the chapter.

Chapter summary

- Clinical practice and decision making draws upon science and the scientific method but is not a straightforward process. An important issue to consider is whether science is a fail-safe or sufficient method for exploring all the factors we need to address in human interaction.
- There are issues with the methods we use to gather knowledge about how the world works; not all things are measurable or predictable. In addition to this, the use to which science is put is open to ideological influences and pre-existing philosophical and political positions on topics. This results in some findings being emphasised, and some being ignored.
- Scientific enquiry takes place in the real world of politics and vested interests. Even if we have sure and certain knowledge, the way we think may distort the application of that knowledge without us even being aware of it. There are external pressures and internal thought processes that result in 'messy' thinking.
- Clinical practice often is based on cognitive short-cut thinking and often out of necessity. We are not cold, rational, linear (cause-and-effect) decision makers; we are human and open to human frailty in our decision making. Therefore, we need systems and processes to improve our thinking in practice.

Activities: brief outline answers

Activity 5.2 Critical thinking

The pharmaceutical industry carries out a great deal of research and development into drug treatments for many conditions and spends billions of dollars on this activity. They therefore need a return on their products to justify continued investment. However, Dr Ben Goldacre (2008) points out that many drug trials are not registered and so we don't know how many trials show negative results. This means we may have incomplete data to compare when judging the usefulness of treatments. He also discusses the 'research' that underpins homeopathic practice and argues that it is selective and bases itself on trials that are too small to show true effects.

Activity 5.4 Decision making

You may have seen a patient who is breathing rapidly (over 25 breaths per minute), who looks pale, and whose lips look blue. You decide to administer oxygen. Some of the information you need for this will have been other clinical signs (e.g. consciousness level) and information given to you by a member of the health-care team (for example, the patient has a history of heart failure). You may also have attended courses in recognising life-threatening emergencies which taught you the airway, breathing, circulation mnemonic as steps to take in reaching decisions. If you review Figure 5.1, you may consider that as time lapse to treatment is crucial you may have relied on system-aided judgements, discussion with peers and, of course, intuitive judgements based on past knowledge and experience. To improve your learning and decision making you may later undertake a critical reflection on the episode using a reflective model to uncover your knowledge and decision-making process.

Activity 5.5 Critical thinking

In the case of the patient with abdominal pain, time is quite short and there are many cues to attend to. This may draw upon our intuitive thinking to enable the complex decisions required to be done quickly, but in addition some analytical thinking can be exercised before the next patient is seen. An issue is that confirmation bias may come to the fore in the analytical thinking as there is not much time to check initial conclusions.

In the case of the MMR vaccine, analytical thinking can be used as this is routine and relatively simple and the public nature of the vaccine has meant that a good deal of literature has been published on the subject. You may have had special education on the subject to bring yourself up to date on the issues. The decision is a week away so there is plenty of time to check all the factors, including the mother's concerns, in a calm reasoned manner. However, being analytical and excluding the need for intuitive thinking may lead us into missing a vital cue because we already know beforehand what the course of action is and fall into the cognitive bias of 'anchoring', whereby the MMR is the overriding fact being considered to the exclusion of other potential health issues (for example, the child's nutritional state).

Further reading

Groopman, J (2008) *How Doctors Think.* New York: Houghton Mifflin.

A very readable text with case studies which neatly illustrate errors in thinking. Although written from the perspective of a doctor, it applies equally to nurses.

Morrall, P (2009) *Sociology and Health.* London: Routledge.

Chapter 3, Science, is a good overview of the sociological debates over the status of scientific knowledge.

Standing, M (2013*) Clinical Judgement and Decision Making for Nursing Students,* 2nd edn. London: SAGE Publications.

A core text covering these issues in much more detail.

Useful websites

www.badscience.net

Dr Ben Goldacre's site examining poor research practice and also the activities of CAMs.

http://io9.com/5974468/the-most-common-cognitive-biases-that-prevent-you-from-being-rational

Discusses common cognitive biases.

Chapter 6
Leadership

```
    ～～～      NMC Standards for Pre-registration Nursing Education
```

This chapter will address the following competencies:

Domain 1: Professional values
4. All nurses must work in partnership with service users, carers, families, groups, communities and organisations. They must manage risk, and promote health and wellbeing while aiming to empower choices that promote self-care and safety.

Domain 3: Nursing practice and decision making
10. All nurses must evaluate their care to improve clinical decision-making, quality and outcomes, using a range of methods, amending the plan of care, where necessary, and communicating changes to others.

Domain 4: Leadership, management and team working
1. All nurses must act as change agents and provide leadership through quality improvement and service development to enhance people's wellbeing and experiences of healthcare.
2. All nurses must be able to identify priorities and manage time and resources effectively to ensure the quality of care is maintained or enhanced.
3. All nurses must be self-aware and recognise how their own values, principles and assumptions may affect their practice. They must maintain their own personal and professional development, learning from experience, through supervision, feedback, reflection and evaluation.

Chapter aims

After reading this chapter, you will be able to:

- understand the policies and context in which nurses have to work as leaders;
- understand leadership in relation to care quality issues in the NHS;
- consider the various theoretical, sociological and psychological approaches that explain what leadership is;
- differentiate between team working and working in a group.

Introduction

The theme of leadership along with management and team working is covered elsewhere in a plethora of books and journal articles, a few of which are listed in the further reading list at the end of this chapter. Rather than going back over well-worked ground, this chapter will examine leadership and management in the wider context in which nurses in the UK NHS operate and will explore how psychology and sociology underpin leadership and management issues. It will then consider how good leadership affects patients' experience, and explore the following argument:

> *although (leadership) is a key area for development, of equal, if not greater importance, is the **need for NHS organisations to create the conditions, which support and enhance new models of leadership** [my emphasis]. Unless this occurs, there is a danger that large numbers of staff will become frustrated at the lack of progress and change, and leadership will simply become another management 'fad' that has failed to have a lasting impact on the NHS.*
> (Hewison and Griffiths, 2004, p. 471)

We need to try to examine the personal troubles that nurses and patients experience, e.g. low morale and poor-quality care in the light of public issues, e.g. the cost of health and social care, and suboptimal care, in terms of the structural transformations in society. These transformations include reform(s) of the NHS such as the impact of the Health and Social Care Act 2012, processes including managerialism, ageing populations resulting in increasing demands on services, geographical mobility and diversity of the make-up of households, in order to put issues of leadership into some sort of social context. This is necessary to enable nurses to understand more fully, and hopefully begin to deal with, the current and future issues of our times.

Leadership policy

Nurses have been called upon to exercise leadership in the health service (e.g. see Hewison and Griffiths, 2004; **http://www.leadershipacademy.nhs.uk**). The document *Making a Difference* (Department of Health, 1999) outlined a leadership role for nurses, emphasising the need for better leadership skills within a wider NHS leadership programme. It was hoped that a new career framework and introduction of nurse, midwife and health visitor consultants would provide a stronger focus for *clinical* leadership. There was a recognition that more emphasis was needed on leadership development, particularly for sisters and charge nurses. This is reflected in the Nursing and Midwifery Council (NMC) (2010) *Standards for Pre-registration Nursing Education*, which state: *All nurses must act as change agents and provide leadership through quality improvement and service development to enhance people's wellbeing and experiences of healthcare* (competence 1 of this domain).

However, the tone of the standards implies a locally focused, clinically based idea of leadership and change. This is implicit when phrases such as quality improvement, service development and risk management are used. These all have specific meanings focused on improving the quality of care for the patient within the UK NHS. The above mention of the 'change agent role', which calls for the enhancement of well-being and experiences of healthcare, could be interpreted to suggest an *outward* population-looking attitude to address national and international health issues that impact on population well-being.

In addition to Department of Health strategies and the NMC standards, the Royal College of Nursing (RCN) offers a variety of leadership courses aimed at enhancing practice and *influencing health and social care policy at local or national level* – note that this is not explicitly at international level, which may be an important omission from an internationalist perspective.

Finally, the NHS has established a healthcare leadership model which can be found at the Leadership Academy website (**http://www.leadershipacademy.nhs.uk**). This model has nine dimensions:

1. leading with care;
2. sharing the vision;
3. influencing for results;
4. engaging the team;
5. evaluating information;
6. inspiring shared purpose;
7. connecting our service;
8. holding to account;
9. developing capability.

These are supported by a self-assessment tool and a 360° feedback tool which is designed to provide other people's perceptions of your leadership abilities and behaviour.

Activity 6.1   *Research and evidence-based practice*

The NHS Leadership Qualities Framework (LQF) was developed for the NHS and set the standard for outstanding leadership in the service. Dennis and Dennis (2006) argue it was a 'traits' approach to understanding leadership as it describes the qualities expected of existing and aspiring leaders. 'Traits' approaches focus on developing individuals rather than the organisations they work in. The healthcare leadership model follows on from the LQF and instead of 15 qualities it has nine dimensions of leadership qualities and behaviours. Again, though, it is a traits approach focusing on the individual. The nature of the organisation nurses work in is not explicitly addressed through this model.

Go to the website and access this page: **http://www.leadershipacademy.nhs.uk/ resources/healthcare-leadership-model**.

Write down what the nine qualities are. You may wish to reflect on: (1) how they apply to you; and (2) if you can see evidence of them in the clinical environment.

continued . . . .

There are other frameworks and models describing the skills and behaviours required of leaders:

- the Medical Leadership Competency Framework;
- the World Class Commissioning Competencies;
- Foundation Trust competencies;
- the Knowledge and Skills Framework.

As this activity is based on your own experience and observations, there is no outline answer at the end of the chapter.

Activity 6.2   *Reflection*

The five factor personality traits test: go to: **www.bbc.co.uk/science/humanbody/mind/ surveys/personality/index.shtml**.

Or search on the BBC website (**www.bbc.co.uk**) for 'big personality test'.

Take the test yourself. Now consider the results: how well do they reflect what you understand about yourself?

As this activity is based on your own experience and observations, there is no outline answer at the end of the chapter.

The conclusion is that you will be expected to undertake a form of leadership in your everyday role as a registered nurse. However, a focus on individual development in this manner is an example of what Hewison and Griffiths (2004) are arguing, i.e. the need for NHS organisations to pay attention not only to the qualities that nurse leaders may have but also to the nature of the organisation in which they work. The most skilled, motivated, competent leader may become frustrated if the organisation does not support the changes required to improve care.

Context: leadership in the public sector

A point to bear in mind about leadership theory is that the literature only really emerged after 1945. Even then, it appeared predominantly in the USA, and applied mostly to the corporate private sector (Parkin, 2010). Therefore, we have to be very careful in applying the theories and concepts to clinical nursing and public-sector organisations. In the private sector, there are various technical skills involved in exercising leadership and management, including:

- financial accounting;
- project management;
- marketing;
- human resources and staff development;
- strategic development.

However, most nurses working in healthcare organisations are rarely involved in these activities. It is not until they move from the clinical role to healthcare management that they undertake these skills. This is not to rule out the exercising of these skills entirely, but they would be based around limited, small projects and budgets. Marketing, of course, is an entirely different activity that is rarely, if at all, addressed by nurses.

Nurses are primarily called to assess, plan, implement and evaluate patient healthcare needs as their primary role. They will do so using their own experience, expert opinion, research evidence, case studies, family and patient input. So, there may be a difference between *clinical* leadership at this level and *managerial* leadership. We will return to this idea later in this chapter.

A key difference between the private and public sector is, of course, that the latter is 'not for profit'. Strategic vision is thus not about research and development for new products to open up new markets based on cost and quality. Strategic vision includes efficiency, effectiveness and high-quality patient experience. Public-sector health issues have focused on the need to provide care, compassion, dignity and cleanliness. These are not commodities as such and cannot be developed and tested. The measures of success do not focus only on the finances; there are multiple 'non-financial' measures. Thus the measure of successful *clinical* leadership, e.g. a patient receiving kindness and compassion, may not show up on the measures that *managerial* leadership requires, e.g. cost.

Thus there is a challenge for clinical nurse leadership in a public-sector organisation. This means that some private-sector skills and outcomes do not apply in the same manner, and the goals and priorities may differ from those charged with managing services.

However, there is pressure to treat public-sector healthcare provision as if it were a private-sector business. Many countries have a mixture of private-sector provision alongside their public provision and this formed the basis for the arguments within the Health and Social Care Act 2012. This introduced the concept of 'any willing provider' allowing 'for profit' organisations, such as Capita, Serco and Virgin. It also allows charities and social enterprises to bid for NHS contracts. This reform of the NHS has run into political trouble in the context of funding pressures on the NHS (Appleby, 2013; Goodman, 2014), and it is likely that further changes may be forthcoming.

We therefore have to ask what patients want from a healthcare system as well as what society is willing to pay for. One answer is to apply the idea of 'public value' – i.e. what is the public getting for its money?

Shareholder dividend is one measure of *private* value, share prices another, but what may be *public* value? This is harder to define.

Chapman (2003) identifies the following characteristics that indicate public value is being added by an organisation:

- The level of service provision is improved.
- The quality of service is increased, particularly in treating all recipients with respect.
- The equity or fairness with which the service is delivered is increased.
- The service provision is sustainable and takes into consideration the needs of future generations.
- The provision of the service is done in a way that is consistent with the expectations of a liberal civic society.
- The service provision enhances the level of trust between government and citizens.

These look like laudable aims, but how do we know we have achieved them? Questions need to be asked about who will measure whether these issues are successful.

Mulgan (2006) and Chapman (2003) suggest that public-sector leadership is best expressed when it is fully involved in the lived experience of the community which it serves. In other words, nurses will have to be fully engaged with their patients, listening to their requirements, negotiating their needs and advocating their positions. Recent high-profile failures in care services in the UK are expressions of just the opposite. *Clinical* leadership may be about meeting those aims for increasing public value but not necessarily meeting the aims set out by managerial and financial targets.

Activity 6.3 — *Critical thinking*

If nurses cannot provide shareholder value, if they cannot increase the hospital's profits, if they cannot therefore increase private value, how can nurses work towards increasing *public* value?

What indicators of care quality are there that nurses can use to show public value? In other words, how does the public know that nurses are giving them a good deal for the money spent on them?

You might want to consider whether the financial bottom line should always be the last arbiter of a quality public service. Sandel (2012) suggests that, in recent decades, market values such as always looking to the 'bottom line' have been applied in almost every aspect of life: healthcare and medicine, education, government, law, art, sports, even family life and personal relations. He wishes us to consider: is this always appropriate?

An outline answer to this activity is given at the end of the chapter.

The current context of NHS working

While the NHS healthcare leadership model outlines the personal qualities required for effective leadership it does not, of course, examine the context in which this leadership has to operate.

Finding out what this context is is a complex matter as this depends partly on who you ask – NHS staff, patients and/or families. As we are focusing on nursing leadership in the context of issues around poor-quality care (clinical leadership), we will look at clues about the context from the nurses' and patients' perspectives.

Activity 6.4   *Research and evidence-based practice*

Where will you find information on patients' experience of the NHS?

An outline answer to this activity is given at the end of the chapter.

The NHS has conducted an 11th annual survey of NHS staff in which almost 416,000 staff were asked about their experiences. The results of the 2013 survey were published at **http://www. nhsstaffsurveys.com**. The survey was designed around four pledges derived from the NHS Constitution (Department of Health, 2009) which in part form the *espoused* (i.e. what we say) social context in which staff work. The statements about what the NHS says it will do are shown below.

NHS Constitution pledges

- Pledge 1: To provide all staff with clear roles and responsibilities and rewarding jobs for teams and individuals that make a difference to patients, their families and carers, and to communities.
- Pledge 2: To provide all staff with personal development plans, access to appropriate training for their jobs and the support of line management to succeed.
- Pledge 3: To provide support and opportunities for staff to maintain their health, well-being and safety.
- Pledge 4: To engage staff in decisions that affect them and the services they provide, individually, through representative organisations and through local partnership working arrangements. All staff will be empowered to put forward ways to deliver better and safer services for patients and their families.

These pledges are in the form they were written for the 2009 version of the NHS Constitution. A post-survey edition of the constitution (2010) can be found at **www.dh.gov.uk/en/ Publicationsandstatistics/Publications/PublicationsPolicyAndGuidance/DH_093419**

The 2013 survey (**http://www.nhsstaffsurveys.com**) found in relation to pledge 4, 'Engaging staff in decisions that affect them', the following.

Trust management

Eighty-two per cent of staff said they could identify who the senior managers are in their organisation (up from 81 per cent in 2012), but only 30 per cent felt that their managers involve staff in important decisions. Just over one-third of staff felt that communication between managers and staff is effective (36 per cent) and just over a quarter (28 per cent) reported that senior managers act on feedback from staff.

Improving the way we work

The proportion of staff saying they are able to make suggestions on how they could improve the work of their team or department has remained stable (75 per cent, compared with 74 per cent in 2012) and 70 per cent felt that they have frequent opportunities to show initiative in their role (compared with 69 per cent in 2012).

Staff as advocates

Over half (58 per cent) of all staff would recommend their organisation as a place to work (up from 55 per cent in 2012). Staff in ambulance trusts were the least likely to recommend their organisation as a place to work (36 per cent), with acute staff being the most likely (60 per cent).

Staff motivation

Fifty-three per cent (52 per cent in 2012) of all staff indicated that they often or always look forward to going to work. Two-thirds were often or always enthusiastic about their jobs (69 per cent) and 75 per cent of staff said that time passed by quickly when they were working.

Key finding 11 was that 38.6 per cent claimed work-related stress in the past 12 months.

The RCN reported on the 2013 survey (**http://www.rcn.org.uk/newsevents/news/article/uk/staff_survey_highlights_serious_cracks_in_the_nhs**) and states:

> *Only 30 per cent of staff think there are enough staff to enable them to do their jobs properly and 82 per cent of nurses continue to work extra hours. 68 per cent of staff have attended work while not being well enough to perform their duties in the last three months alone.*

Dr Peter Carter, Chief Executive and General Secretary of the RCN, said:

> *During the last year, the NHS and its staff have faced a great deal of change, scrutiny and pressure. Clearly, nurses and other staff are working hard to ensure that patient care is delivered. However, it is simply not sustainable to have staff stretched too thinly and working beyond breaking point.*
> (**http://www.rcn.org.uk/newsevents/news/article/uk/staff_survey_highlights_serious_cracks_in_the_nhs**)

The RCN also undertook a staff survey in 2013 (response rate of 14 per cent, just over 9,000 useable responses) and found:

- *The nursing workforce across all health care settings are regularly working high levels of overtime – and usually unpaid. Over half (56 per cent) report working extra hours on every shift or several shifts a week while two thirds (66 per cent) are working over 2 hours overtime every week. Our survey respondents told us that workload and stress are their main personal concerns, ranked above all other worries about their and their families' health, their own job security and that of their partner or household income and expenditure.*

- *. . . further evidence of heavy workloads, work pressure and staffing levels. Respondents working in all health care settings report decreasing staffing levels with half reporting that the number of registered nurses have fallen and a third reporting the number of health care assistants (HCAs) and health care support workers (HSWs) has fallen in the previous 12 months. In addition, one third report that staffing levels for both registered nurses and HCAs/HSWs have fallen in their workplace.* (RCN employment survey 2013: **http://www.rcn.org.uk**)

The results of the surveys are mixed and need interpretation. One could cherry pick the results to show better or worse staff feelings about working in the NHS; with that caveat in mind there are still serious issues that need addressing.

Clinical leadership in this context, then, is a nurse facing inadequate staffing levels in a Trust that is facing efficiency savings with possible job cuts in the pipeline, a managerial leadership issue. The exercise of leadership takes place in a real social world where *perceptions* as well as reality impact on how nurses think about themselves, their work and their organisations (Royal College of Nursing, 2011b).

However, it is not all doom and gloom. There are instances where nurses are making a real difference to the quality of patient care, and it is necessary to learn from such cases to understand the critical factors that turn things around. One of those critical factors may be the organisation's trust and support for change and innovation that come from nursing staff. Also, it may well be the case that nurses can take the personal qualities invested in themselves (as perhaps outlined in the NHS LQF) to make the most of the opportunities presented to them. The example of Salford NHS Trust is probably worth a more detailed examination than can be given here (see case study below).

Case study

The Salford NHS Trust considered that to improve the quality of care the focus had to be on patient safety. The Trust introduced a number of measures based on a corporate strategy to save 1,000 lives and to reduce harm by 50 per cent. Patient safety was thus the driver for improving quality care. An important aspect of the strategy was to see nurses as the spine of the organisation. The view was that they should hold equal responsibility and accountability alongside medics and service management. In addition, they argued that nursing is the 'go to' profession because they, alongside other professional groups, know what the problems are and how to solve them. Leadership in this context was one aspect of the overall strategy (which included staff involvement and a clear exposition of values) which illustrated 'board to ward' commitment to organisational change rather than just relying on individual teams to force change through.
(http://www.cqc.org.uk/content/quality-care-nationwide)

What does 'leadership' mean for you?

Leadership as a concept can be difficult to grasp. The word is often used interchangeably with 'management' but they do not mean quite the same thing. In the USA, and increasingly also in the UK, the word 'leadership' has particular connotations. It is seen as 'a good thing'; it is 'romanticised'; and 'we need more of it' – and there is the idea of the 'heroic leader' who, if appointed, will 'sort things out'. This notion of the heroic leader is challenged by the King's Fund (2011) report into leadership, clearly stating: *no more heroes*. The King's Fund report argues for a notion of leadership that is *shared, distributed and adaptive* rather than reliance on a chief executive. You will read about the lack of leadership in NHS organisations as being one reason for the issues of poor-quality care.

Activity 6.5   *Critical thinking*

What do you understand by the two words, 'leadership' and 'management'?

Make a list under each heading. Then discuss this list with a colleague and/or your mentor in practice.

An outline answer to this activity is given at the end of the chapter.

As already stated, there are many texts on leadership and we refer you to further reading on this. However, for our purposes we may consider an overview of leadership and management theory as the following.

- Theories based on 'person' (traits). These theories seek to understand it from the position of the individual person and may ask: what attributes, qualities or characteristics are needed in a leader? This looks for the attributes of the 'great man'. This underpins many NHS leadership development programmes.
- Action-centred leadership theory is a way of understanding leadership, developed by John Adair (1973), who asks us to consider that it is more than just about the individual. The team and the nature of the task, as well as the individual, have to be studied to understand fully how leadership operates.
- Behavioural theory. Leadership can be studied by the behaviours and styles that leaders adopt. For example, authoritarian (just do it), democratic (how shall we do it?) or laissez-faire ('doing it' emerges with little direction) styles of leadership.
- Formal/informal leadership can be exercised by formally appointed people and/or arise through informal processes, from people who may not have a formal title of authority but who exercise leadership through their experience, drive and initiative.
- Transactional/transformational theory. Managers transact (they get the job done) while leaders transform (they focus on vision and developing people) (Bach and Ellis, 2015).
- Distributed or shared leadership models (King's Fund): less emphasis on the 'boss' accepting followers is important.

> ## Concept summary: Leadership theory based on person and behaviour
>
> Kouzes and Posner (2011) suggest the following are common to successful leaders:
>
> - Challenge the process – first, find a process that you believe needs to be improved the most.
> - Inspire a shared vision – next, share your vision in words that can be understood by your followers.
> - Enable others to act – give them the tools and methods to solve the problem.
> - Model the way – when the process gets tough, get your hands dirty. A boss tells others what to do; a leader shows that it can be done.
> - Encourage the heart – share the glory with your followers' hearts, while keeping the pains within your own.

Nurses as leaders

Cunningham and Kitson (2000a, b) evaluated the RCN clinical leadership course and suggest that there are five key areas in which leadership needs developing in individual nurses. So, to help us think about how we exercise leadership it is useful to consider these five areas as a guide to personal development:

1. Managing self: Who are you? What are your strengths and weaknesses? What motivates you? Are you emotionally intelligent? What is your default ego state? What is your relationship to the organisation in which you work? What are your hopes, dreams and ambitions? What are your personal values?
2. Managing the team: What theories do you hold about working with people? What makes for good team working? What personal core skills are required for team working? What assumptions do you have about how people work? What power dynamics are you aware of?
3. Patient-centred care: What does this mean in detail? What behaviour and attitudes do you possess that hinder or foster this? Is there a difference between the theory and practice of patient-centred care?
4. Networking: Who is in your network? What tools do you use to network? What skills are required for networking? What does networking mean in nursing? Why is networking valuable?
5. Political awareness: What are the policy drivers affecting you and your work? Who are the key players? How can you affect decisions? At what level should you operate?

As a student nurse you will be focusing a great deal on point 3, patient-centred care, and you will be introduced to point 2 probably in your third year. Many of your activities and reflections will also help you with point 1 (managing self). Networking and political awareness may then be addressed upon registration (or they may not). You may have already started networking. Facebook is a vehicle for social networking and it may also be used for professional networking, as may sites such as **http://uk.linkedin.com**. We suggest that these are very important skills to have and reflect that a lack of them results in staff being unable to control and understand their working environments.

Again, we see in this approach elements of trait/personal development (points 1 and 2), but points 4 and 5 indicate the need for an awareness of wider organisational issues, as Hewison and Griffiths argue should occur. Point 5 particularly suggests that leadership development, i.e. political awareness, ought to address wider organisational issues as well as developing yourself.

Professional networking

Many professionals are now using internet-based sites such as Linkedin (**http://uk.linkedin. com**) to make contact and share ideas with others, not only of their own profession but also of related professions. Look out for professional nursing networks such as the International Council of Nurses' student network: **www.icn.ch/networks/student-network**.

For Facebook as a professional interest group: see **www.facebook.com/groups/NursingSCC**.

For a Twitter network see: **#nurchat** for twice-weekly discussions.

We may also need to consider that leadership operates at three levels:

1. micro (patient);
2. meso (ward/unit/clinical team, hospital, clinic);
3. macro (health service, national and international).

Therefore, you may wish to see your developing skills in leading happening at these three levels. Upon registration you may concentrate on the first, you will have been introduced to the second and as you gain experience and skills you may operate at the third. The micro level will require your personal skill development, but the meso and macro level will require organisational changes which a clinical leader may only *influence*.

Leadership vs management – the same or different?

Activity 6.6   *Team working*

If nurses are not leading projects or accounting for financial spending, what does exercising *clinical leadership* mean? There is a view that there are competing ideas about what clinical leadership is, what professional values and assumptions it is based on and how this

---

contrasts with notions of *managerial leadership*, which has very different assumptions and values about how healthcare is delivered (Edmonstone, 2009).

After reading Edmonstone's paper, discuss these two questions with two or three peers.

1. What is meant by *clinical* leadership as opposed to managerial leadership?
2. Discuss the notion of the 'disconnected hierarchy'.

Write the various responses of individuals from the group on to a flip chart.

An outline answer to this activity is given at the end of the chapter.

Bennis and Goldsmith (2003) argued:

> *There is a profound difference between management and leadership, and both are important. To manage means to bring about, to accomplish, to have charge of or responsibility for, to conduct. Leadership is influencing, guiding in a direction, course, action, opinion. The distinction is crucial.*
> (cited in Bogle, 2009, p. 159)

They go on to specify the following distinctions between the two.

- The manager administers, the leader innovates.
- The manager is a copy, the leader is an original.
- The manager focuses on systems and structures, the leader focuses on people.
- The manager relies on control, the leader inspires trust.
- The manager has a short-range view, the leader has a long-range perspective.
- The manager has his or her eye always on the bottom line, the leader has his or her eye on the horizon.
- The manager imitates, the leader originates.
- The manager accepts the status quo, the leader challenges it.

It is useful to reflect on how this leadership, thus defined, is exercised in clinical practice. Consider the exercise of innovation, originality, people focus, trust, long-termism, horizon thinking, originality and challenge. To be able to do this requires authority to act in this regard in an organisation that supports and encourages such leadership qualities, as Hewison and Griffiths point out. The *Making a Difference* document (Department of Health, 1999) focuses on strengthening leadership, especially at sister and charge nurse level; however, to what extent are nurses at this level empowered to lead rather than manage more efficiently? Leadership requires the power to act proactively rather than responding to policies, procedures and guidelines within a context of bureaucratic managerialism. Risk management, clinical governance and quality improvement are arguably aspects of efficient management rather than the exercise of leadership.

Bogle (2009) discusses his vision of corporate leadership, which incorporates both aspects of managing and leadership, but he writes from the perspective of the chief executive officer. Sisters and charge nurses operate at middle-management level and this is often characterised as having responsibility without power to affect real change at the organisational (NHS Trust) and public policy level. Nurses may well defer to medics, Trust managers and government ministers in all local and national healthcare policy matters unless there is structural change, as exemplified at Salford but not at Mid Staffs, being undertaken in the organisations in which they work.

Thus, leadership may be about vision and change, but the structure of an organisation means a focus on management. Nurses may be in relatively powerless positions to affect policy (Bishop, 2009) as cultural influences affect working practices:

> *[N]urses . . . tend not to own any power in policy making terms . . . gender stereotyping, medical dominance and inadequate professional leadership . . . conspire to keep us in places where others want us.*
> (Bishop, 2009, p. xv)

In the next section, we examine how the external context of management practices affects the internal reasoning of individual nurses which then may affect patient care.

Rationality, managerialism and the lifeworld of compassionate care

The nursing care experiences of older people in the UK have been much reported in the national and international press. Reasons for that poor quality of care in hospitals often focus on the 'culture' of organisations, as well as on individual failings. However, discussions about culture change are partial explanations without a deeper analysis of how cultures and leadership operate in sociopolitical contexts which characterise nurses' 'lifeworlds' (Goodman, 2014). Therefore the solutions may not address wider determinants of care, such as risk governance, managerialism, instrumental rationality and, of course, staffing and skill mix. Instead, organisations may be exhorted to change their cultures, without addressing these wider determinants and thus poor care practices may continue to occur. If targets are abolished, this may still leave a layer of managerialist thinking. This impacts on education because students, who are 'working and learning', experience occupational socialisation through immersion in the *lifeworlds* of their clinical colleagues.

Rationality

To get from public issues of social, and organisational, structures to the personal troubles of patients experiencing indignity there is a need to apply a little sociological imagination (Wright Mills, 1959). The suggestion is that modern society is characterised by a *rational* approach (Weber, 1992) to issues including the management of risk, and it is this *instrumental rationality* (*Zweckrational*) that has unintended consequences for the care experience. Weber's theory of 'rationalisation' suggests that modern societies become increasingly rational and bureaucratic, whereby social life becomes more and more prone to scientific analysis, measurement, bureaucratic control and the application of 'instrumental rationality' to social problems and issues. *Instrumental rationality* is a mode of thought and action that identifies problems and works directly towards their solution, often focusing on the most efficient and cost-effective methods of achieving certain ends. It may not stop to ask what those ends should be, or what effect efficiency and cost-effectiveness have on human relationships. This is Sandel's (2012) point regarding using market principles in every area of social life. A falls risk assessment could be seen as an efficient and cost-effective measure to reduce the number of falls, and it is part of the overall instrumental rational approach to risk management. Actually constraining a patient's mobility to prevent a fall may be *rational,* but it may not be *human.* Discharging a patient back home according to the tenets of efficiency and effectiveness of hospital services may be rational, but it is not always human.

Instrumental rationality in the context of funding gaps in the NHS results in the prioritisation of the bottom line and financial efficiencies. Adverse events, such as falls, not only cause human suffering but perhaps more importantly for those charged with running hospitals and care homes, also cost money and therefore must be avoided.

The health service over the past few decades has increasingly sought to eradicate uncertainties in care, and to control its costs, by the application of practices of regulation and surveillance – protocols, monitoring, targets, audits, evidence-based practice and performance measures. This sets up a dichotomy for care staff in that they deal with 'the human' in direct contact, but at the same time are expected to complete myriad managerial diktats, many of which are about controlling risk. These tools, on their own, do not automatically result in indignity. However they are part of a wider organisational and social mind set that can reduce patients into categories and numbers and a 'data set'. This process can 'infect' nurses' mind sets or 'lifeworlds'.

Lifeworld

Nurses and their patients inhabit a 'lifeworld' (*Lebenswelt*) of intersubjective perceptions and meanings (Husserl, 1936). It is experienced as that which is 'self-evident' and 'taken for granted'. The lifeworld has some 'objective' truth, is always 'there', and is a shared foundation for our experiences as nurses and patients. This includes the rules, goals, values and meaning of our shared social and nursing actions. You might experience this as 'just the way things are' and often as accepting of the cultural assumptions of the clinical experience and workplace practices without critical thought or reflection. A common aspect of the lifeworld for the patient on admission is assuming the role of the patient, leaving personhood behind, as we accept name tags and often subservient roles. The lifeworld of nursing includes assumed values of care rather than profit as the goal of work.

However, this 'taken for granted' human lifeworld of nursing is open to 'colonisation' by other values and attitudes such as rationality (Habermas, 1984), i.e. that rationality can become a taken-for-granted aspect of nursing. Social roles on the ward and its lifeworld are based upon the actions of its members and also the requirements of wider social structures of management, hierarchy and, what Habermas considered, 'oppressive' systems. These requirements, e.g. managerialism, manifest in the need to control, record and risk assess everything, and can overwhelm and penetrate nurses' lifeworld – colonise it – so that nurses then take on this rationality 'as a given'.

This might result in cognitive dissonance as nurses struggle to reconcile humanistic care with the technico-rationality of medical and managerial requirements. This may result in feelings of disempowerment, rendering nurses unable to criticise or posit an alternative set of caring practices or contexts. For Habermas, the colonisation of the lifeworld by the instrumental rationality of bureaucracies is a key aspect for the analysis of modern societies. When nurses uncritically take on board the tenets of bureaucratic rationality, or the managerial goals of efficiency, effectiveness and increasingly profit, their humanistic lifeworlds are thus 'colonised'. This is another aspect of the theory–practice gap, in that students may learn their practice based on humanistic values but then, via the resolution of any cognitive dissonance they might feel when confronted by the *reality* of clinical practice (Curtis, 2013), may come to practice *instrumentally* in a rational, but not necessarily human, way.

So what is this managerialism that is liable to 'colonise our lifeworld'?

Managerialism has been understood as both a process and an ideology (Enteman, 1993; Preston, 2001). Its nature and growing influence in both the private and public sector have been described elsewhere (Hood, 1991; Enteman, 1993; Drucker, 1994; Hoopes, 2003; Lees et al., 2013). A defining characteristic is the application of *scientific and rational* means to the achievement of certain organisational goals. Hood (1991) referred to 'new public management' which, since the 1980s, was aimed at reforming the public sector through the application of market mechanisms and a focus on outcomes and efficiency. Preston (2001b) argues *it is a belief in a strategic approach . . . making objective and deterministic claims about the nature of our social and professional practices.* Fitzsimons (1999) wrote that managerialism is a form of *instrumental reasoning* in which efficiency is a defining goal, *regardless of the value* of the activity itself. In the current context of the NHS, a focus on patient safety, efficiency and effectiveness by management might be characteristic of this frame of mind.

Hillman et al. (2013) explain the management of risk in organisations using the idea of 'governmentality' as a form of managerialism. This involves individuals implicating themselves in their own 'governance', in the internal control of themselves. This is a focus on how the mechanisms, tools and techniques for managing risks shape human conduct. This is about *control of self*, getting nurses to *self-police* through the acceptance and internalisation of certain ideas. This is achieved through the acceptance by nurses of certain discourses – in this case, a discourse of managerialism, risk aversion and risk management through rational action.

The result of these processes may be that face-to-face interaction with patients is compromised in favour of the collection of more abstract factors and information that are seen as increasing risk for patients, and the need to control it. The plethora of data collected to manage patients' risk better may have a tendency to leave little room or time for human caring. In this manner we might not be able to pay attention to the *soft intelligence* or *soft metrics* (Cottrill and Gary, 2006), e.g. a relative's story or a cold cup of tea, that is flagging issues with care practices. Belatedly, the

NHS is waking up to the need to listen to patients who are well able to provide feedback on their care experiences. Ashley (2013) reported that Dr Martin McShane, director of long-term conditions for NHS England, acknowledged at the 2013 Future for Health conference that there is a need for a *radical new approach* in the NHS. This 'radical' approach turns out to be listening to patients (!) through a *people's panel* (Ashley, 2013). The people's panel put across messages such as the need for doctors to spend time talking to 'people' rather than 'patients'.

Not listening to people, not picking up on 'soft metrics', results in cultures of care that lack humanity (Hillman et al., 2013). Indeed, the Francis reports (2010, 2013) highlighted a target-driven management culture as a causative factor in the poor care of patients. This target-driven management culture is what *colonises the lifeworld of nursing*. To address compassionate care, organisations should consider *flexible person centred risk taking* (Edinburgh Napier University and NHS Lothian, 2012). Smith (2012) suggests, however, that despite nurses still wanting to give compassionate care, systems need to be in place to allow them to do so. The current context has seen the dilution of the role of the ward sister by a complex system of managers and mentors (Cornwell et al., 2013); therefore this key role for the development of values and support of staff has fallen victim to the wider process of risk aversion and managerial control. If clinical leadership (Edmonstone, 2009) is to be exercised, there is a need for clinicians to be free and supported to provide it.

So, leadership in certain contexts means challenging taken-for-granted practices and seeing beyond one's personal development as the only answer to better care. Next, we examine team work, another concept seen as important for improving the quality of care for patients.

Team working

Team working is a theme that appears a good deal in the literature, the focus being on ensuring good team work to improve patient outcomes. There are descriptions about what makes a team, what holds teams back from working effectively, how we develop a team and what the proper role for team members may be. However, we also need to think critically about our teams in practice. Is team working myth or reality in clinical practice? We suggest that culture, organisational development and notions of what leadership and management may be will affect how a team performs, whether it actually is a team or merely a group. As MacGregor argued: *most teams are not teams at all, but merely collections of individual relationships with the boss. Each individual vying with the others for power, prestige and position* (cited in Sargent, 2006, p. 295).

This comment followed Miller's (1999) observation that: *some health care teams exist in name only, demonstrating little evidence of collaborative working underpinned by shared goals* (cited in Goodman, 2011d, p. 36).

Chase (1995) had previously examined team working in critical care environments and observed two parallel hierarchies consisting of medics and nurses. The suggestion here is that clinical teams may divide along professional lines and are not teams at all but are merely groups. This idea related to Edmonstone's (2009) idea of two 'disconnected hierarchies' in healthcare – clinicians and managers.

Activity 6.7 — *Team working*

Discuss the difference between what makes an effective team and how this differs from being a 'group'. Clark (1997) lists the characteristics of a team. Do you see any parallels with what you have identified as the characteristics of an effective team?

The characteristics of a 'team' (Clark, 1997):

- collaboration – nurses working together to share ideas, resources, questions, the evidence base;
- shared goal or task – this is clearly identified as ensuring a patient's 'care pathway' is complete;
- mutual accountability – nurses call each other to account for actions and omissions; it is 'everyone's business';
- interdependence – nurses cannot undertake the work without other people supporting them; others need nurses to fulfil their role;
- commitment – 'we will see this through day after day, week after week';
- personal growth – who we are and how we grow as professionals and as people are important to each other;
- synergy – the coming together of ideas, which results in innovation and change;
- cooperation – 'we all play our part'.

As this is group work you will come to your own conclusion about the teams you work in, so there is no outline answer for this activity.

Katzenbach and Smith (1993) differentiate between what constitutes a true team and what is just a working group (Table 6.1).

Within nursing teams and their relationship with other professions (e.g. medics) there are various barriers to team development. These barriers may come from issues of gender and sex role stereotyping (male doctors, female nurses), status and class. Other barriers could include separate professional education and separate lines of management. We have already noted the difference between managerial leadership and clinical leadership, and this may result in a business culture vs a care culture, i.e. public-sector value vs private-sector value.

In addition, teams need to develop and grow as they sort out their 'group dynamics' – how individuals relate to each other.

Tuckman (1965) outlined a typology for group dynamics and argued that teams went through various stages of development. The implication here is that if a team gets stuck at one stage they will not get to optimum performance.

Tuckman's 'stage theory' was based on research he conducted on team dynamics. He believed as is a common belief today that these stages are inevitable in order for a team to grow to the point

True teams	Working groups
True teams share leadership roles as they see fit	Working groups have a strong and clearly focused leader
True teams take mutual, collective accountability	Working groups take individual accountability
True teams create specific team objectives that they deliver themselves	Working groups' objectives are imposed, mandated, granted and/or the same as the broader organisational mission
True teams deliver collective products/ outcomes	Working groups deliver individual products/outcomes
True teams encourage open-ended discussion and active problem-solving meetings	Working groups run efficient meetings
True teams measure performance directly by assessing collective products/outcomes	Working groups measure effectivenesss indirectly by their influence on others

Table 6.1: True teams vs working groups (based on the work of Katzenbach and Smith, 1993)

where they are functioning effectively together and delivering high-quality results. In 1977, Tuckman, jointly with Mary Ann Jensen, added a fifth stage to the existing four stages: *adjourning*. The adjourning stage is when the team is completing the current project. They will be joining other teams and moving on to other work in the near future. For a high-performing team, the end of a project brings on feelings of sadness as the team members have effectively become as one and now are going their separate ways.

The five stages are:

1. forming;
2. storming;
3. norming;
4. performing;
5. adjourning.

Many clinical teams within professions are characterised by individuals coming and going at regular intervals. If Tuckman is correct, we may be faced with the fact of established teams who are performing and having to face a constant stream of new members. These new members may have already progressed through the other stages and this may constantly disrupt the performance of the team. Stability of team membership then would be key to keep it at the performing stage. Students joining clinical teams will experience the forming/storming/ norming stages and will have to do so very quickly. Clinical leaders thus would have to ensure a quick and safe passage through these stages to ensure their teams stay performing. Transformational leadership may be the most appropriate way of doing this, although it does have its critics (Hutchinson and Jackson, 2013), based around its inability to deal with the power context in which it is supposed to operate. See Bach and Ellis (2015, pp. 98–99) for an overview of this important concept.

Team role theory

A key part of the development process which it is suggested a leader has to facilitate is the recognition that each team member may have a specific team role, a set of attitudes and aptitudes that they bring. Belbin suggested various team roles which, if brought together, will support effective team working.

Consider the various roles outlined by Belbin (2003) and reflect: if teams did not have, for example, a 'completer finisher', what this would mean for team performance? (See **www.belbin.com/ rte.asp?id=8**.)

To apply team role theory to nursing teams assumes something about what the nature of nursing actually is. Consider whether nursing teams require all of the roles Belbin outlines.

Chapter summary

- Leadership has become an important concept in the NHS. It rests alongside management as a key aspect of nursing work.
- The exercise of leadership, and what it actually means, varies considerably and is affected by both external social and policy issues as well as the individual characteristics possessed by people.
- A good deal of effort is being spent on developing individuals so that they can fulfil leadership and management functions, but whether any of this does any good in terms of direct patient outcomes is a complex question.
- Hewison and Griffiths point out the need for organisations and their cultures to change to allow certain qualities and practices to emerge. This theme is echoed in a good deal of the literature on leadership.
- Leadership cannot be understood without placing it in some political context. How clinical teams work together, patient expectations and NHS reforms all impact on nurses and their ability to manage and lead.
- Patients and families are being encouraged to express their needs and wants, and herein lies a problem. The public want something from a public service that may not be able to be delivered – in an era of rising expectations and increasing demands, how nurses work within the larger NHS machine will not always be in their control.
- Effective clinical leadership will need every nurse to examine some of these core ideas to enable the planning and delivery of safe, effective and dignified care.

Activities: brief outline answers

Activity 6.3 Critical thinking

This is a complex question. It may be useful to divide this into measurable outcomes (such as mortality rates, pain relief) and subjective measures (such as privacy, dignity, comfort). This really is a question that nursing leaders will clarify in their work.

Activity 6.4 Research and evidence-based practice

Go to the following websites:

www.dh.gov.uk/en/Publicationsandstatistics/PublishedSurvey/NationalsurveyofNHSpatients/index.htm

http://cqc.org.uk

To access results for a Trust, enter a postcode or organisation name, go to the Trust page, then go to the middle tab, 'Reports and surveys about this organisation', and scroll down to 'What people said about this trust'.

Survey data are available for the following surveys:

- 2009 Outpatient survey – acute and acute specialist trusts;
- 2010 Survey of women's experiences of maternity services – acute trusts;
- 2010 Acute adult inpatient survey – acute and acute specialist trusts;
- 2011 Community mental health survey – mental health, care trusts and primary care trusts providing mental health services.

Activity 6.5 Critical thinking

Bogle (2009, p. 159) suggested the following distinctive definitions of the terms 'leadership' and 'management':

- The manager administers, the leader innovates.
- The manager is a copy, the leader is an original.
- The manager focuses on systems and structure, the leader focuses on people.
- The manager relies on control, the leader inspires trust.

Compare this with the answers you came up with in discussion with your colleagues.

Activity 6.6 Team working

There are many definitions of clinical leadership, but it may be useful to differentiate it from managerial leadership. Clinical leadership is about patient-focused and peer-focused activities, being knowledgeable about clinical practice, accessing and using the evidence base, leading innovations in care and fostering good interprofessional relationships. It is about putting patients at the core of activities and advocating for their interests over and above the interests of the organisation. You may wish to add to this.

Further reading

Bach, S and Ellis, P (2015) *Leadership, Management and Team Working in Nursing*, 2nd edn. London: SAGE Publications.

This book explores students' current perceptions and concerns, giving practical guidance for immediate challenges the new nurse will face: team working, delegation, conflict management and negotiation. It then considers staff development and motivation, mentoring, supervising and creating a learning environment.

Later chapters explore more complex aspects such as management theory, recruitment, risk management and managing change.

Goodman, B and Clemow, R (2010) *Nursing and Collaborative Practice*. Chapter 5, Teamwork. Exeter: Learning Matters.

Useful websites

http://www.leadershipacademy.nhs.uk

The home site of the NHS leadership academy.

www.nursingleadership.org.uk/index.php

Go to the above site, find the 'self-assessment tests' tab and attempt the 'Your leadership style' and 'Your team role' tests.

https://www.academia.edu/4710241/Leadership_and_Management_in_Nursing_-a_critical_approach

Online teaching document on leadership.

Chapter 7
Death, stress and resilience

NMC Standards for Pre-registration Nursing Education

This chapter will address the following competencies:

Domain 2: Communication and interpersonal skills

5. All nurses must use therapeutic principles to engage, maintain and, where appropriate, disengage from professional caring relationships, and must always respect professional boundaries.

Domain 3: Nursing practice and decision making

4.2. **Adult nurses** must recognise and respond to the changing needs of adults, families and carers during terminal illness. They must be aware of how treatment goals and service users' choices may change at different stages of progressive illness, loss and bereavement.

Chapter aims

After reading this chapter, you will be able to:

- discuss theories of death and dying;
- understand bereavement and grieving processes;
- explore the role of the nurse in supporting people who are dying and the bereaved;
- consider and explore your own views on death and dying;
- consider how to 'look after yourself' to create personal ways of dealing with death and loss and stress.

Introduction

It is both a cliché and truism to state that death affects everyone whether we work in healthcare or not, and so we need to think about what this means both for ourselves and for our patients. We will begin with an overview of the social nature of death before exploring it from a more individual and personal perspective. An understanding of the social, and sociological, nature of death helps to challenge assumptions and taken-for-granted beliefs; nurses will be better able to deal with the various understandings and meanings people attach to death and dying if they realise that dying is not a purely personal and biological event. We will also discuss the psychology of death and bereavement, including stress and coping with challenging events, and will conclude by considering ways in which we can improve our well-being.

Durkheim and suicide

A classic sociological treatise on death remains the work of Emile Durkheim, whose investigations into 'suicide' (1970, first published in 1897) emphasised the need to understand the social context of death, which not only gives it its meaning to individuals, but also affects the manner of death. He introduced the notion of 'social forces' acting upon individuals, arguing that it was the 'force' of their integration of Catholics into their own society that results in a form of social control. This control, he theorised, led to lower suicide death rates among Catholics compared to Protestant populations. Thus, death is both social and an individual event.

This Durkheimian perspective takes a social position, i.e. membership of the Catholic Church, and relates it to an individual's psychological motivation, the decision not to commit suicide, suggesting that what might look like a decision made with free will may be a result of accident of birthplace and cultural upbringing. This takes us back to considering the agency–structure arguments raised throughout this book. To what degree are we exercising free will, our own personal agency, even in matters of death and dying?

Death and society

Death can be understood as a physical event, when the body can no longer function. However, this would be only a partial understanding. An additional way to understand death is the idea of 'social death'. Death is a social event; it is socially organised, overseen by various rituals, meanings and definitions (Kastenbaum, 2001). Societies' norms, values and laws construct the dying process, the meaning of death and the death event itself; for example, the rituals that are enacted. When we say death is socially 'organised', we are referring to the ways that society makes death happen in various ways and that an individual's passing may not be just the result of a biological event, such as a viral infection. The following discussion on road traffic accidents is an example of what we mean by society 'organising' death. The word 'organising' does not, of course, refer to a committee consciously planning death, although in countries past and present that is almost exactly what happens. The 'organisation' refers to the patterns and structures of how we go about living our lives, including how we think about and go about our dying. This then suggests that if society changes its patterns of living and its social structures, we would see a change in the patterns of dying.

In the UK the medical profession takes control of death, having the legal power to define who is dead and when the moment of death happens. It is almost as if death does not occur unless a medic says it does. Atul Gawande (2014) suggests that, in the USA, and also in the UK, we have medicalised death both in terms of location – we die in hospitals, not our homes – and in terms of treatment. He suggests that doctors often forget the well-being of the patient in their anxiety to do everything medically possible to prolong life.

In applying the sociological imagination to death we come to understand that this very 'personal trouble' is also a public issue in that there are culturally appropriate ways of dying and responses to death that exist in each society and over time. Hence, death has different meanings to different people. It is not just the event itself but the process of dying that is also social in nature. Nurses play an important part in the way society controls death and dying. Palliative care principles have become an important skill set for many professional nurses working, for example, in hospices.

Society also organises death by producing the conditions under which many people die. Different historical eras produce differing patterns of death, an obvious example being the relative non-existence of road traffic deaths in eras when the only means of transport was the horse. This is not to say that people did not die under the wheels of wagons or by being thrown off horses – in that sense, 'road' deaths did occur. The difference is in technology, high-speed impacts, scale and perhaps severity of death and injuries as part of everyday life. Chapter 4 outlined the social structural effects on death rates in relation to health inequalities.

Activity 7.1 — *Research and evidence-based practice*

How many people, do you think, are killed or injured on Britain's roads in the course of a year?

See: **www.rospa.com**.

An outline answer to this activity is given at the end of the chapter.

The death system

Kastenbaum (2001) discussed the concept of the 'death system', i.e. *the interpersonal, sociocultural, and symbolic network through which an individual's relationship to mortality is mediated by his or her society* (Kastenbaum, 2001, p. 66). Through this concept, Kastenbaum seeks to move death from a purely individual concern to a larger context, understanding the role of death and dying in the maintenance and change of the social order.

The death system has several components. First, it involves people, including those who earn a living from death, e.g. palliative care nurses, coroners, funeral directors, florists, insurers. The second component is place, i.e. hospital, hospice, home, mortuaries; third is times, such as Armistice Day (11 November) or Good Friday. Finally, objects and symbols – a diverse category that includes mourning clothes, last rites and aspects of language. A society's death system has several functions:

1. warning about and predicting death;
2. caring for the dying;

3. disposing of the dead;
4. social consolidation after death and adjusting to new circumstances;
5. making sense of death;
6. sanctioning killing.

Death systems evolve over time in response to changing circumstances. A study of death systems reveals the varying ways in which cultures deal with this certainty and demonstrates that what seems normal and natural in one culture is not so in another.

Nurses can be seen to play a more or less active part in each of the first five of the six functions above. Nurses are therefore integral to the death system, for example, performing last offices (function 3) and post-bereavement information and guidance (function 4). The sixth function, 'sanctioning killing', really only applies to politicians and the military, although the topic of euthanasia and assisted suicide regularly comes up for debate.

The medicalisation of death

In Chapter 2, we looked at Illich's (1975) critique of the medical profession, and the medicalisation of everyday life extends to the medicalisation of death. Medics' intervention has become the source of the primary definition and processing of death in many advanced countries as part of their 'death systems'. The few remaining indigenous cultures that exist will 'do' death differently, and have very different death systems.

Morrall suggests (2009) that medical oversight, definition and control of death result in an idea of the *ideal type* of death, which is *a death by natural causes at the end of healthy life* and is related to the idea of the medic working (heroically?) to achieve this. This also relates then to an idea of the 'untimely death', or the idea of a *good death* (Kellehear, 1990), which is a socially regulated death that accords with society's values, and in the UK's current context this means that it needs to be overseen by the medical profession. It is now necessary for someone to die of 'something', hopefully medically defined, and die 'somewhere', usually in an institutional facility of some sort. For detailed information on end-of-life care in the UK, see Public Health England (2013). Hospital remains the most common place of death, but there is an increase in home and hospice deaths. This is partly attributed to the National End of Life Care programme (Public Health England, 2013).

If we consider that a professional group (medics) defines, manages and oversees death we might want to consider whether, as individuals or as members of less powerful professional groups (nurses), this organisation of death is the only or best way to do it. Medics have critiqued their own handling and management of death (Gawande, 2014); some have raised the question about unnecessary prolongation and medical intervention for patients that they would not want for themselves (Murray, 2012). Healthcare professionals who understand the limitations of modern medicine may thus opt out of life-prolonging treatment. Murray (2012) argues that the best death can be the least medicated, allowing the patient to die peacefully at home. Society's values change and the debate over assisted suicide, including the role of the Swiss clinic Dignitas, illustrates how the social regulation of death is a dynamic process which then affects what we count as a 'good death'.

Lord Falconer's Assisted Dying Bill was debated in parliament in November 2014. The argument is that the law should allow terminally ill, mentally competent adults to request life-ending medication from a doctor. The patient, or should we say, person, would have the right to self-administer that medication should he or she choose to do so. According to the campaign group Dignity in Dying, a YouGov poll found 73 per cent of adults in England and Wales support the Bill (**http://www.dignityindying.org.uk/assisted-dying/lord-falconers-assisted-dying-bill**).

Organising death

An earlier description of how society 'organises' death was outlined by Glaser and Strauss (1965) through their construct: *awareness contexts*. This describes the process of negotiation that occurred between patients, families and healthcare staff to address the dying process and experience (see concept summary box below).

Glaser and Strauss's *closed awareness* negotiation context may accord with Western values (and male values?) but ethnic, class and age differences may not fit easily into this context. Some people would value open awareness over closed awareness and vice versa.

Sudnow (1967) argued that the patients' social status and condition influenced things such as resuscitation decisions, the type and extent of medical interventions and even how quickly death is pronounced. Children would get different attention from alcoholics or the elderly. Timmermans, following up this work later (1998), argued that changes in practice, technology and protocols acted 'merely' to justify decisions already made by staff about who to resuscitate. Sudnow's work suggests an *inequalities in death* concept in which social factors such as age and drink and drug use lead to less effort on behalf of medical staff. It also suggest that assessments of the moral worth of patients might be at play. Hill (2010) appears to provide a measure of support to these arguments, stopping far short however of suggesting that the moral judgements engaged in by healthcare staff result in death. Hill argues that moral judgement of patients is pervasive, occurring not only in *egregious and criminal* cases, but also in everyday situations in which appraisals of patients' social worth and culpability are routine. The full impact of moral judgement on healthcare relationships, patient mortality, decisions to resuscitate and clinicians' own well-being is as yet unknown. The paucity of attention to moral judgement represents a blind spot that requires examination in far more depth. The prevalence and dynamics of moral judgement in healthcare are also unknown.

Concept summary: Glaser and Strauss's 'awareness contexts'

- Closed awareness: the patient is not aware of dying, but others are.
- Suspected awareness: the patient thinks s/he is dying and tries to elicit this information from others.
- Mutual pretence: both sides know the situation but no one admits or discusses it.
- Open awareness: the dying person also knows and it is openly discussed.

These contexts form the backdrop of discussion around how the death should be handled.

Wittenberg-Lyles et al. (2009) examined hospice healthcare staff's discussions about the patient's care. They suggest that there is a 'backstage' and a 'frontstage' discussion. Frontstage is where the healthcare team discuss and negotiate with the patient and family. Backstage occurs without them; it involves communication between the healthcare team that patients and families don't hear and helps in the management of emotions by healthcare staff. Glaser and Strauss's 'awareness contexts' are all frontstage.

Activity 7.2   *Reflection*

Consider a situation in which you have been involved in the care of a dying patient. Can you identify any of the contexts outlined above? Did they occur in order?

As this activity is based on your own experience and reflection, no outline answer is given.

Glaser and Strauss later (1968) also discussed seven critical junctures. These are social phases of the dying process and form part of a *dying career*.

1. the reclassification of a person as healthy to a patient who is dying;
2. family and friends start making emotional and practical preparations for the death;
3. the 'nothing more to do' phase;
4. the final descent;
5. the last hours;
6. the death watch;
7. the death.

This career pathway describes the social process of dying; however, this is an 'ideal type', a *description only*. Many people will not go through this process and nurses will have to be prepared to encounter a wide variety of responses by people and their families to the fact of death and their dying. This description is now quite dated and it may well be the case that it reflected medicalised and controlled death in a different social era. Whether this death career still applies is open to question.

Death denial

As well as developing the well-known stages of dying, Elisabeth Kübler-Ross (1969) thought that Western culture was *death-defying*, that we do not wish to contemplate or openly discuss death, and that we could learn from other (non-Western) cultures. This is a recurrent theme in contemporary literature but has much older roots in philosophy, especially in the work of Epicurus (341–270 BCE). Philippe Ariès (1981) argued that death in the West has become a *shameful event*; his work was based on historical analysis where he argued that Western death is *invisible death*. To support this thesis, Elias (1969, 1982) suggests that Western society is characterised by a civilising process whereby extreme feelings and behaviour get constrained; death in this context then gets 'screened off' as it is too 'messy' to deal with.

Lawton (2000, 2002) discusses the concept of the *unbounded body*. An unbounded body is where the person loses control of bodily functions and fluids. The civilising process (Elias, 1969) and the medicalisation of death result in death being managed away from us in everyday experience and moved to clinical environments. The decision of where to die thus rests on the conditions of unbounded body – that is to say, that as the human body loses control of basic eliminatory functions, for example, we tend to transport the dying physically into clinical environments (hospitals) where we can attend to the cleaning rituals. We have to ask ourselves whether this is always the best answer and whether nurses can support family members in caring for the *unbounded body* (i.e. their loved one!) in places of their own choosing.

Kübler-Ross's criticisms of a *death-defying* West may be a value position, and a question remains why other cultures' views on death may be the right way. Why should openness (open awareness) be favoured above all else? An older study by MacIntosh (1977) suggested that actually patients did not want to know they were dying. However, this is over 30 years ago and patients' views may well have changed.

According to Public Health England (2013), the National End of Life Care Strategy (Department of Health, 2008b) recognised that death is a taboo subject for the majority of people in England. In 2009, the National Council for Palliative Care set up the Dying Matters Coalition to promote public awareness of dying, death and bereavement. The 2010 *British Social Attitudes Survey* (National Centre for Social Research, 2010) found:

- Although 70 per cent of the public say they are comfortable talking about death, most haven't discussed their end-of-life wishes or put plans in place.
- Only 35 per cent of respondents said they have a will. This is down from 39 per cent in 2009. Economic pressure is a possible cause of this decline.
- Fewer than a third (28 per cent) have registered as an organ donor or have a donor card – although the number of organ donations after death has risen by 50 per cent since 2008. More than 1,000 people on the transplant waiting list die each year (NHS Blood and Transplant figures: **http://nhsbtmediaservices.blob.core.windows.net/organ-donation-assets/pdfs/transplants_save_lives.pdf**).
- Only 11 per cent have written their funeral wishes or made a funeral plan.
- Five per cent say they have set out how they would want to be cared for at the end of life if they couldn't make decisions themselves.
- Seven per cent say they would prefer to die in hospital, compared to two-thirds (67 per cent) who would prefer to die at home.

Zimmerman (2007) had suggested that this denial is still contemporary. This 2010 survey suggests it might still be. 'Death denial', our social reticence to discuss the reality of death and dying, is also a feature of palliative care literature and practice, and has been seen as an obstacle to the components of care that constitute a *correct way to die* (Zimmerman, 2007). These 'care components' include open discussions of dying, dying at home, stopping futile treatments, advance care planning and the control of symptoms. The argument here is that denying death prevents these components of care from being enacted. This argument draws upon the US experience, where palliative care contexts differ from the UK, but illustrates again how social processes impact on the dying.

We have to consider the role of nurses in all of this and reflect to what degree nurses are in control or can act as patient and family advocates in this process. Are we a death-denying/defying society, or is it the case that death has been removed from everyday experience?

Bereavement

The use of terms in this area is complicated and tends to overlap, so do not worry if you cannot make precise distinctions. We may define loss as the experience of an absence in an individual's life. This could be the absence of a person, or any important aspect of life. What often follows on from this is grief, which is the emotional response to loss. We also may engage in anticipatory grieving, i.e. the emotional response to an anticipated loss. This may well occur after a poor prognosis has been given to us. Mourning is the behavioural expression of grief and may take various forms. There may well be cultural and religious patterns to mourning that need to be taken into account.

Activity 7.3   *Research and evidence-based practice*

What mourning rituals and practices are carried out by differing ethnic and religious groups? Choose one or two ethnic or religious groups and research mourning rituals and practices. Collate your findings and use them as if you were going to present them to a seminar group. You may wish to do this with a friend, each of you choosing a group and then sharing your findings.

An outline answer to this activity is given at the end of the chapter.

We may define bereavement as a 'period of emotional adjustment that follows the death of a loved one'. The death of a loved one is not the only form of bereavement. The loss of a spouse, a job, health or home may give rise to considerable grief. It is the state of having lost someone or something; this state is characterised by feelings of grief and the expression of these feelings in mourning.

It is important to remember when caring for family members that the period immediately after a death can be a busy one. There will be a lot of practical issues to deal with. After this, there may be a lot more time for grieving, and grief can be a long process. Sensitivity, patience and support are called for.

Grief

We may suggest that the pain of grief is the price we pay for love, the cost of commitment. If we have never given to someone, if no one is ever important to us, if we have not loved, then we may not have grieved either. The time scale for the grieving process varies, averaging 18 months to 2½ years. Loss is a very personal thing and so are reactions to it. A major bereavement shakes confidence in an individual's sense of security: consider long-married couples who have grown their own personal rituals and support systems for each other. When one partner dies, grief can be very isolating. Many older people end up living alone and a sizable minority will feel loneliness. The Campaign to End Loneliness has found that *research over decades has found that a fairly constant proportion (6–13 per cent) of older people feel lonely often or always* (**www.campaigntoend loneliness.org.uk/ loneliness-research**).

The mourning process has been described (Parkes, 1972) as stages but, as with many stage theories, this is not to be taken as a literal or linear approach to understanding human action and reaction. Parkes described four phases:

1. numbness;
2. yearning for the lost one;
3. disorganisation and despair;
4. reorganised behaviour.

Although it may be useful to consider this as a pathway and an 'expected journey', everyone's experience is individual. Stroebe and Schut (1999) suggested that there is no simple progression towards the resolution of one's grief; rather we oscillate between grief and restoration. What this means for care staff is accepting and expecting unpredictability when helping the bereaved.

Bereavement and young people

Death and dying are not the preserve of the older person; they affect the young both as patient and as relative (son, brother, granddaughter) and there will be age-dependent understanding and incomplete understanding of what is occurring.

For children up to 5 years, death may be seen as sleep, as not final or irreversible. The child may be more curious than frightened. Between the ages of 5–9 the idea of death being final is being developed and then around 9 or 10 years the child has some understanding of processes involved and may realise the finality of it all. Note these age ranges make it difficult to assume exactly what children will know at what age. A child's incomplete understanding may lead to difficulties for the child and carers, as the child may expect the person to return. Children may believe that person has intentionally left them, e.g. because they were 'bad'. The death of a sibling may present particular problems because of normal tensions and jealousies between siblings.

Your needs as a student nurse

Dealing with loss and death is a complex business. People are unpredictable and emotional. Responding to loss in others is very demanding and will call upon your stress-coping mechanisms, your personal philosophy and your understanding of what your proper role should be. You yourself are likely to experience loss in your work and in your personal life (if you have not done so already). The next section on stress outlines some issues to consider. You will need to develop and ensure that you have appropriate professional and personal support. You will need to go on a personal journey to explore your own feelings towards, and understandings of, death, loss and bereavement, and how you cope with the resulting stress. Space precludes a discussion of the various ways people have developed to understand death and loss, but we will share a few in the hope that you will find a path suitable for you and those you work with and those you love. The following opinions from Steve Jobs and Irvin Yalom are offered in this spirit.

Case study for reflection: Death is the destination we all share

Steve Jobs (the Chief Executive Officer of Apple, Inc.) gave an address to graduates at Stanford University, California, USA in 2005. It is available online as text and on YouTube. Access this speech and reflect on his view on life, death and the human experience. Find it here: **http://news.stanford.edu/news/2005/june15/jobs-061505.html**.

Irvin Yalom and death anxiety – *Staring into the Sun*

Sorrow enters my heart and I am afraid of death.
(Yalom, 2008, p. 1)

Irvin Yalom draws upon Greek philosophy, existentialism and psychodynamic theory to argue that the knowledge of our own mortality (our *mortal wound*) affects the unconscious mind of every human being.

Every individual unconsciously has to deal with the fact of their own death and some experience of death anxiety. This will require a reconciliation. We have to reconcile ourselves to the facts of our own death. Yalom observes that dealing with death is 'difficult': *You cannot stare straight into the face of the sun or death,* except that we have to do so at some point. Death anxiety is the price we pay for that awareness. To deal with that anxiety we may engage in adaptive or maladaptive coping strategies. These range from denial to avoidance. We invest in wealth, our children, our career, hedonism, cosmetic surgery, religion, drugs, fame, anything but face death. Yalom argues, however, that death anxiety is always there, lurking in the background. He suggests we confront it head on, that we indeed stare into the face of the sun.

There are solutions to our 'existential fears', fears based on the knowledge of our finite existence. These include thinking about certain ideas. The root cause of human misery is our omnipresent fear of death or our denial of the transient nature of existence. Yalom cites the Greek philosopher Epicurus and his reasoning about death as a way of confronting it. Epicurus argued as follows.

1. The soul is mortal and dies with the body, therefore there is no need to fear an afterlife because there is none.
2. Death is nothingness.
3. Symmetry: we have experienced oblivion already and following the briefest of lives we will experience it again.

There is no reason to fear death because our lives and our deaths are mutually exclusive: *Where death is, I am not; where I am, death is not.*

Yalom offers up the idea of rippling, to counter the view that life is ultimately meaningless. We create concentric circles of influence that may affect others for years or even generations. This idea is that to pass on something of ourselves, often without our knowledge, may give meaning to our existence. The implication, then, is to live so that we send out positive rather than negative ripples.

The good life is thus not about duration but about achieving tranquillity (Greek: *ataraxia*). If the goal of life is to lead a tranquil life, then its duration is immaterial. Thus what we are in the here and now is important, not what we possess or what our reputations are. The latter are two goals we may chase at the expense of achieving *ataraxia*.

Epicurus and Yalom are materialists and do not believe in God or gods. They do not dismiss the fear of passing into death, the pain and suffering that result as we go on our way, but death itself is nothing to fear. In a similar way, Buddhists hold to the notion that the root cause of human suffering is our denial of our own transience. To ease this we need to meditate on the meaning of life and death, live in the present and be mindful of the pleasures that life bestows in the here and now. Attempts to ward off death may thwart a more mindful attitude to death and life.

We may say with Epicurus that we agree, that death holds no fear for us, but are we able to deal with our visceral emotions regarding our own mortality? Is rationalising on death enough for us? That is a personal journey we will all have to make.

This is one view. Postmodern theorists would emphasise the fragmentation of social life in which old conceptions (about death) are breaking down and individuals are creating their own identities and meanings of the death experience. Nonetheless, society is ambiguous about death. It sanctions death on a grand scale, sets the conditions in which people die, how they die and how they are pronounced as dead.

Ultimately, the only control individuals have is about how they deal with death anxiety.

Despite the numbers attending churches, mosques and synagogues, we have a paradox in society in that we have become largely secularised in terms of organised religion, at least in the UK, and yet many of us are seeking answers to life in the 'spiritual' gap that science and technology have left behind, through 'new ageism', for example. The messages of the Abrahamic religions, i.e. Christianity, Islam and Judaism, have not been universally accepted or mutually tolerated, and so, with the certainty of our mortality, many try to grasp a new meaning. However, as society has become more individualised and consumerist (Baumann, 2000) and with its value on youth culture, if not youth worship, death has become the new taboo.

Despite the fragmentation of orthodox religions into their fundamentalist and literalist forms, i.e. those who focus on the literal truth of their sacred texts to the exclusion of others, there remain communities of believers in all three Abrahamic religions focused less on interpreting the literal truth and more on core values of community and care. It might be fair to say there is as much a divide between fundamentalist forms of religion and their ecumenical/community/liberal-oriented wings as there is between religion and atheism. You will find meaning in religion, atheism, humanism, Buddhism and philosophy. This search for meaning and community might be protective regarding death anxiety. What we do know is that loneliness and isolation are detrimental to health and well-being. Loneliness kills (Monbiot, 2014; Perry, 2014).

Developing resilience

Death and loss may be stressors. Certain clinical environments are said to be stressful for various reasons. Palliative care settings confront the practitioners daily with the fact of death and loss. However, the resulting pressures that may lead to stress can come at any time and in any clinical setting. We will now examine the relationship between stress, stressors and health, and suggest ways in which we might begin to protect ourselves from health-damaging environments.

To begin to unpick how we may cope with stress we need to understand a little about the mechanisms. To do this we will briefly discuss Hans Selye's general adaptation syndrome (GAS), which focuses on understanding the stressor itself, and then Lazarus and Folkman's (1984) transactional model, in which an imbalance between the perceived situational demands and perceived available coping responses may result in a stress response.

Hans Selye's general adaptation syndrome

The GAS (Selye, 1956) is a three-phase model of stress response, based on the theory that because stress causes long-term chemical changes, it also then results in disease. Our bodies respond biologically to external threats and stressors; the response involves hormone release within the 'fight or flight' stress response. This results in an imbalance which the body tries to restore, and it is this process of restoration that Selye calls GAS. However, the body only has a limited supply of adaptive energy, which declines with continued exposure, resulting in damage to cells and organs.

The general adaptation syndrome and stages of response to stress

1. Alarm: Flight or fight reaction. The arousal hormones (cortisol, adrenaline and noradrenaline) cause high blood pressure and increased heart rate. If this energy is not repeatedly used, then this may cause harm.

2. Resistance: As the stressor is resolved, homeostasis begins to restore balance; arousal is then lower but not normal. There may still be stress as hormones return to normal but you may have reduced defences and energy. If this process is repeated too often with little or no recovery time, this may result in physical health problems.
3. Exhaustion: You have no reserves, the stress has continued, the body's ability to resist is lost as the adaptive energy is gone. This stage may be termed overload, burnout, adrenal fatigue, maladaptation, dysfunction. Stress levels go up and stay up.

We might suggest that for some people working in settings where they lack control, have little autonomy, have high expectations and demands placed upon them and have relatively low income (e.g. care assistants; remember Richard Wilkinson and Kate Pickett's (2010) thesis that relative income, not absolute income, is important for health inequalities), then the continued stress placed upon them depletes their physical resources, resulting in overload and burnout. If this occurs, we can hypothesise that the end result may be poor performance and poor-quality care experienced by patients.

The transactional model of stress

Richard Lazarus and Susan Folkman (1984) suggested that stress results from an *imbalance between demands and resources* and occurs when *pressure exceeds one's perceived ability to cope.*

While Selye focused on physical stress as direct response to a stressor, Lazarus and Folkman suggested that stress management should be about resources and our ability to cope to mediate the stress response.

If we wish to develop an effective stress management programme, the first step is to identify how people go about controlling their stress, and then to identify the intervention methods that focus on how people go about that control.

This interpretation of stress focuses on the transaction between people and their external environment (hence the transactional model). Stress may not be a stressor if the person does not perceive the stressor to be so. Indeed, the stressor may be perceived to be positive or even challenging. If the person possesses or can use adequate coping skills, then stress may not actually result or develop because of the stressor.

If this is the case then we may suggest that people can be taught to manage their stress and cope with their stressors. They may learn to change their perspective of the stressor and thus develop the ability and confidence to improve their lives and handle all types of stressors. This might sound a little like 'positive psychology', shifting the focus on to the individual's perceptions and coping mechanism rather than the structural issues (e.g. low pay, lack of control). It may have the benefit of reducing or ameliorating the perception of threat while not actually removing the source. This could be useful in situations where structural issues (e.g. poor skill mix) cannot be solved.

Concept summary: Lazarus and Folkman's transactional model of stress

There is a 'primary appraisal' (the appraisal of the situation) where we ask: 'Does the situation require a coping response?' Then there is the 'secondary appraisal', where we ask: 'Do I have the resources to cope?' If coping is required but the resources are not available, stress is experienced. Then there may be a 'reappraisal', when stressors and responses are reappraised to reduce the experience of stress.

Primary appraisal (of the situation)

1. An 'event' occurs, the appraisal may result in no coping required or
2. An 'event' occurs, the appraisal may mean a coping mechanism is required
Is there perception of harm?
A challenge?
A threat?

Secondary appraisal (of the situation)

Do I have the resources to respond?	If not, then I experience stress
Can I cope?	

Figure 7.1: Diagram to explain Lazarus and Folkman's transactional theory of stress

People cope with stress in various ways. Lazarus and Folkman divided this into two categories.

1. Problem-focused coping: here I may focus on appraising the problem and finding solutions.
2. Emotion-focused coping: my feelings towards the stressors are managed.

Problem-focused coping is more effective as it deals directly with the problem and may solve it, thus removing the source of stress. However, in reality we may suggest everybody uses a combination of the two.

In addition, we may adopt adaptive (positive) or maladaptive (negative) coping mechanisms when trying to address our stressors.

The health realisation/innate health model

The health realisation/innate health model of stress (Banks, 1998) is also founded on the idea that stress does not necessarily follow the presence of a potential stressor. Instead of focusing on the individual's appraisal of so-called stressors in relation to his or her own coping skills, as the transactional model does, the health realisation model focuses on the nature of thought, stating that it is ultimately a person's thought processes that determine the response to potentially stressful external circumstances. In this model, stress results from appraising ourself and our circumstances through a mental filter of insecurity and negativity, whereas a feeling of well-being results from approaching the world with a 'quiet mind'.

This model proposes that helping stressed individuals understand the nature of thought – especially providing them with the ability to recognise when they are in the grip of insecure thinking, disengage from it and access natural positive feelings – will reduce their stress.

Activity 7.4   *Critical thinking*

Under two headings list adaptive and maladaptive coping mechanisms, i.e. those activities that will help or, if not hinder, merely mask the problem.

An outline answer to this activity is given at the end of the chapter.

It has also been suggested that there are personality variables, e.g. Kobasa's (1979) idea of one's personal *hardiness*, that will help or hinder our stress response. If you have a high degree of *self-efficacy* (Bandura, 1977), you are more likely to see threats as challenges to be overcome; you have a lot of energy to bring to your activities, as well as commitment to see things through. This is because you have belief in your own capacities – you believe you can organise your abilities and resources and that you can follow this through with action to achieve your own ends.

A point for student nurses and their mentors to reflect on is: how do we develop this sense of self-efficacy in practice? Is this a personality issue, i.e. relying on the personality of the student, and/or an organisational issue? Chapter 6 suggested that there is a need for organisational change as well as leadership development.

Burnout stress syndrome

Freudenburger (1974) suggested that *burnout stress syndrome* was common in the caring professions. Tillett (2003) argued that doctors and other healthcare professionals experience higher rates of psychological morbidity (e.g. anxiety, depression, suicide) than the general population. The reason may be pressures of clinical work but this may also be 'helping profession syndrome'. This is when a person unconsciously chooses a career in healthcare as a response to his or her own personal vulnerability, i.e. helping the 'patient within'. McVicar (2003), Collins (2006) and Riahi (2011) suggest that stress is still a serious issue for nurses. The effects of stress and burnout include: emotional exhaustion, depersonalisation, i.e. treating 'clients/patients' in an impersonal way and diminished feelings of personal accomplishment, accompanied by cynicism. If we think back to the actions undertaken by staff towards patients at Mid Staffs, we may consider that stress and burnout might have played a role. It is interesting to consider whether the application of a tool such as the Maslach's Burnout Inventory – General Survey (Maslach and Jackson, 1986) might have predicted high levels of staff stress in this case.

Sources of stress come from external pressures, organisation issues, such as bullying management and poorly trained co-workers, as well as from patient issues such as their emotional journey and their dying experience. Selye points to physical effects, while Lazarus and Folkman focus on coping with and adapting to stressors. Your 'hardiness' and self-efficacy may be useful in protecting you from the demands placed upon you, but it might be asking too much of individuals if they work in poorly led and badly managed organisations. Your ability to affect the organisation at this stage in your career will be limited, but you may be able to do something to improve your resilience to life's challenges. The next section addresses the idea of well-being and how you may be able to increase this in your life.

Five ways to well-being

In 2008 the New Economics Foundation was asked to review the work of over 400 scientists to establish an evidence-based set of actions to improve well-being (**http://www.nationalaccountsofwellbeing. org/learn/related/five-ways-start.html**). This set of actions could be used by individuals in their daily lives to help to reduce stress, improve coping mechanisms or build personal capacity (such as self-efficacy).

The five ways are as follows.

1. Connect – with the people around you, family, friends, colleagues, neighbours. Time should be seen as investment in these people as the cornerstone of your life.
2. Be active – take physical exercise (walking, cycling), find something you like and that suits your level of mobility.
3. Take notice – develop mindfulness of things around you, be curious, note the seasons changing, savour the moment, reflect on experiences and appreciate what you have.
4. Keep learning – try something new, rediscover an old interest, go on a course, learn new skills, set yourself challenges.
5. Give – do something for a friend, commit random acts of kindness, join a group, volunteer.

Aked and Thompson argue:

> *The Five Ways to Wellbeing was developed based on evidence relating to individuals' behaviour. If individuals change their behaviour so as to incorporate more Five-Ways-type activities into their day-to-day lives, the empirical evidence suggests that their subjective wellbeing should improve.*
> (Aked and Thompson, 2011, p. 36)

The five ways are in early development in terms of providing evidence of outcomes for well-being, as Aked and Thompson again argue:

> *Whilst the Five Ways to Wellbeing themselves are evidence-based, in future there will be a need for robust evaluations of their implementation and application. To put it plainly, whilst [a] survey . . . tells us something about the ways in which the Five Ways to Wellbeing can be used, it tells us nothing about which uses are more or less effective in improving wellbeing.*
> (Aked and Thompson, 2011, p. 37)

Despite the current lack of evidence for improved well-being (the concept itself might be difficult to measure), the five ways at least provide a positive set of actions, adaptive coping mechanisms, to deal with stress and prevent burnout.

However, a purely personal response to well-being and stress coping without addressing the structural causes (e.g. unemployment, poverty) is not sufficient. Nurses, as discussed in Chapter 6, have to work at various levels, individual and social, to improve working lives for themselves and to improve the quality of the patient experience.

There is a lot of literature on stress and burnout in healthcare – social factors such as gender and socioeconomic status may play a part, as may age, in terms of coping strategies adopted by people. However, what works for you is part of your personal self-development and should be seen as an important aspect of your professional learning.

Chapter summary

- Death is a 'social event' and not a purely biological occurrence for the individual. Society manages and controls death through the 'death system' it constructs, which nurses are a part of.
- A major part of the UK's death system is medicalised, i.e. controlled by medics, but this is changing. Patient and healthcare professionals often have unacknowledged social roles for dealing with death and dying.
- Death, loss and bereavement are stressful life events but are inevitable aspects of life which need to be confronted. Bereavement is a complex process which will have varying individual responses.
- Healthcare practice is stressful and nurses may suffer burnout, which may lead to poor care.
- Dealing with stress involves understanding its effects and developing positive coping mechanisms.
- Positive life actions towards well-being may help to build personal resilience.

Activities: brief outline answers

Activity 7.1. Research and evidence-based practice

Britain has one of the best road safety records in Europe and the world. Despite massive increases in traffic over the last few decades, the number of people killed on our roads has fallen from around 5,500 per year in the mid-1980s to well under 2,000 in 2010. However, this still means that around five people die on Britain's roads every day. Reported road casualties in Britain in 2010 (Department for Transport, 2011) are as follows:

- killed: 1,850;
- seriously injured: 22,660;
- slightly injured: 184,138;
- all: 208,648.

Activity 7.3 Research and evidence-based practice

There are many resources you can access for information about mourning rituals and practices, but here is one example:

> *Sikhs cremate people when they die. When someone seems about to die their family will come to their bedside and say Sukhmani (the Hymn of Peace). The dying person tries to reply Waheguru. The dead body is washed and then dressed in traditional Sikh clothing.*
> (**http://www.bbc.co.uk/schools/gcsebitesize/rs/death/sikhdeathritesrev2.shtml**)

Activity 7.4. Critical thinking

- Adaptive: talking things over with friends, counselling, physical activity, confronting the problem and seeking solutions.
- Maladaptive: keeping it to oneself, drink, drugs and smoking, denial of the issues.

Further reading

Costello, J (2006) Dying well: nurses' experiences of 'good and bad' deaths in hospital. *Journal of Advanced Nursing*, 54 (5): 594–601.

This article suggests that the death experience is related to the degree to which nurses have the ability of control over the dying process.

Gawande, A (2014) *Being Mortal: Illness, Medicine and What Matters in the End.* Canada: Doubleday.

A book that explores whether we have exalted longevity over what makes life worth living and considers attitudes towards the old.

Howarth, G (2007) *Death and Dying: A Sociological Introduction.* Bristol: Polity Press.

This book provides a comprehensive discussion of the key topics in death and dying, using material from cross-national and cross-cultural perspectives. It carefully addresses questions about social attitudes which will be useful for nurses.

Kübler-Ross, E (2009) *On Death and Dying: What the Dying Have to Teach Doctors, Nurses, Clergy and Their Own Families*, 4th edn. Abingdon: Routledge.

The updated version of this classic text was written when the author was dying.

Useful websites

www.crusebereavementcare.org.uk

Cruse Bereavement Care.

http://www.neweconomics.org/issues/entry/well-being

The New Economics Foundation's Five Ways to Well-being project.

www.nhs.uk/conditions/stress/Pages/Introduction.aspx

The NHS Choices site for stress.

www.apa.org/helpcenter/road-resilience.aspx

Information about recent strategies for developing resilience.

Chapter 8
Maternity and children's nursing

Chapter aims

By the end of this chapter you will be able to:

- discuss the social meaning of pregnancy and childbirth;
- understand the arguments about the choice of place of birth;

- explore the meaning of parenting;
- describe the stages of child development;
- discuss social attitudes to children and families.

Introduction

The Nursing and Midwifery Council (NMC) outlines that nurses from all fields of practice have to address fields other than their own. What follows here are some psychosocial issues in the field of children's nursing and maternity care, which will be useful to all nurses who will need to have a broad understanding of any person who might come into their care irrespective of their field of practice. An omission here is a detailed discussion of fatherhood or paternity. These subjects are not covered in depth in textbooks or in the literature, and this may illustrate the gendered nature and assumptions about the nature of family, childbirth and child care. That being said, the arguments around the meaning and social role of motherhood can be equally applied to fatherhood.

Maternity care

The social meaning of pregnancy and childbirth

The 'medicalisation' of childbirth during the latter half of the twentieth century (Oakley, 1979, 1980, 1984; Hunt and Symonds, 1995) has seen birth transferred into the care of obstetricians and hospital midwives. However, this trend has been challenged by a move back towards more home births under the supervision of midwives. Whether care is under the supervision of midwives or medical staff, the main trend has been the professionalisation of birth, removing it from the care of professionally unqualified women.

There is now a recognition that non-healthcare staff have a role to play, with the introduction of the 'doula', a Greek word meaning woman servant or caregiver, an experienced woman giving emotional and practical support to women before, during and after birth (**www.doula.org.uk**). However, it would be rare indeed for birth to be overseen by a doula alone. Both the Royal College of Midwives and the Royal College of Obstetricians and Gynaecologists support home births where there are no expected complications.

Maternity care (pregnancy and childbirth) is bounded by medical understandings of the management of pregnancy and questions over what is a safe birth (i.e. in hospital, overseen by medics and obstetricians) but this is contested by, for example, the radical midwives' view. You can find these contrasting views on the various organisations' websites, e.g. the Association of Radical Midwives, at **www.midwifery.org.uk**; the National Childbirth Trust, at **www.nct.org.uk/about-nct**. The Royal College of Midwives also runs a 'campaign for normal birth' (Royal College of Midwives, 2011a).

| Activity 8.1 | Research and evidence-based practice |

What percentage of women choose a home birth? Discuss the reasons why home birth is or is not chosen. See **www.patient.co.uk/doctor/Booking-Criteria-and-Home-Delivery.htm**

Consider your opinions about the best place to have a baby. What are they and what are they based on?

Consider your opinions about the role of fathers around childbirth. Again, what is this based on?

As the answers to this activity will be based on the relevant statistics for the year you are looking up, and on your own thoughts and reflections, no outline answer is given at the end of the chapter.

The Association of Radical Midwives began in 1976 when student midwives felt that there was increasing (and, by implication, too much) medicalisation and intervention in maternity care. As a result, a journal, *Midwifery Matters*, is now available to support the objectives of advocating for women's active participation in care and to explore alternatives to (medical) care. The issue that began this process in the 1970s was the common practice of the artificial rupture of membranes around a woman's due date. This was not felt to be a necessary intervention and exemplified the medicalisation of maternity care.

Concerns about safety underpin many discussions about childbirth. Women die giving birth, particularly if we consider all women across the globe, and the reduction of such deaths has been highlighted as one of the eight Millennium Development Goals (United Nations, 2012). The good news from the United Nations is that most deaths are avoidable. To address this issue, the UK has published detailed information on maternal deaths since the 1950s. The first report was the *Report on Confidential Enquiries into Maternal Deaths in England and Wales 1952–1954* (Ministry of Health, 1957), and an up-to-date report has been produced every 3 years. The latest one, *Saving Mothers' Lives*, was published in March 2011 (Centre for Maternal and Child Enquiries, 2011). In the first half of the twentieth century, the UK maternal mortality rate was around 50 per 100,000; the rate is now about 13.4 per 100,000 (Drife, 2005). The Centre for Maternal and Child Enquiries takes over from the Confidential Enquiry into Maternal and Child Health and is due to produce a ninth report.

Globally there is steady progress in saving mothers' lives; there has been a 45 per cent reduction in maternal deaths since 1990 (World Health Organization, 2014). The reasons for those deaths include pre-existing conditions such as diabetes, HIV, malaria and obesity. These account for one in four maternal deaths. Severe bleeding during pregnancy and childbirth account for one in four deaths. There are of course wide differentials across regions of the globe. A 15-year-old girl in sub-Saharan Africa faces about a one in 40 risk of dying in pregnancy and childbirth compared to a one in 3,300 lifetime risk for Europeans.

So, while it is undoubtedly the case that maternal deaths have been reduced in the UK over the last 50 years as a result of early diagnosis and effective treatment of obstetric complications

(Drife, 2005), the degree of medical intervention at all stages of pregnancy remains an issue, as does the question of who should be the lead professional involved. Pregnancy can thus be understood to be a normal and natural process requiring care from non-medical staff in non-medical settings unless risk assessment suggests that medical complications and co-morbidities decree otherwise. The concern over maternal deaths may have been a driver to medicalise the pregnancy and birth experience. However, is this concern always justified?

The National Institute for Health and Care Excellence (NICE) issued guidance in 2014 suggesting many more babies could be born outside hospital. This guidance applies to England and Wales. About 700,000 babies are born each year in the two countries; nine out of ten are born in doctor-led obstetric units in hospital. There are higher rates of medical intervention for those giving birth in hospital than those at home, but why this is so is not known. It is suggested that midwife-led settings have better outcomes for mothers than traditional hospital-based units (NICE, 2014).

We may reflect that this is about society's and individuals' control over our bodies – who has control, who exercises control, where that control is exercised. Then there are issues over the experience of pregnancy and whether 'pathologies' related to pregnancy are individual and organic, or social, or a complicated mix of all these factors.

What this means is that we have to consider as taken for granted assumptions about childbirth, ante- and postnatal care, and consider whether medical definitions actually serve all women well. This requires a critical look at the evidence base for safe birth and ante-/postnatal care. This is assisted by guidelines found on the websites of NICE and the two Royal Colleges (Midwives, and Obstetricians and Gynaecologists), which are listed at the end of this chapter.

A more recent and pressing issue is that even maternity care in hospital is being compromised by issues around adequate staffing and concerns about the quality of care (Royal College of Midwives, 2011b), with the issues being rising demand, massive midwife shortages and an ageing workforce.

Other current issues for maternity services outlined by the Royal College of Midwives (2011c) are:

- the involvement of fathers in maternity care ('the invisible parent');
- a fall in the number of home births;
- the increase in caesarean section rates, and what this means for women;
- women on low incomes getting a poor deal from maternity services;
- budget cuts and gaps in resources.

Pregnancy and childbirth exist within a culture that has differing ideas about what the whole process of childbearing means for women, for their babies and for men. How maternity services are delivered by society is based on contrasting ideas but has been dominated by medical definitions of the experience. Issues around social structure and inequalities in health also impact on the birth experience. Activity 8.2 will help you understand the global inequalities in health around maternal mortality.

Activity 8.2   *Research and evidence-based practice*

Go to the United Nations Millennium Development Goals website: **www.un.org/ millenniumgoals**. Find the maternal health link. How many women die annually from complications during childbirth? What percentage of that number will be in developing countries? How many children per year are left motherless?

You may also wish to visit Hans Rosling's Gapminder site, at **www.gapminder.org**, and explore the maternal mortality data.

An outline answer to this activity is given at the end of the chapter.

Many of the issues touched on in this chapter so far could be seen to be based on the idea of 'woman-centred care' (see concept summary box below), which it is suggested has developed out of a concern over the medicalisation of pregnancy and childbirth, and a male-centric/ scientific philosophy.

Concept summary: Woman-centred care

'Woman-centred care' is the term used to describe a philosophy of maternity care that gives priority to the wishes and needs of the user, and emphasises the importance of informed choice, continuity of care, user involvement, clinical effectiveness, responsiveness and accessibility. The fundamental principles of woman-centred care ensure:

- A focus on pregnancy and childbirth as the start of family life, not just as isolated clinical episodes, that takes full account of the meanings and values each woman brings to her experience of motherhood.
- Women are equal partners in the planning and delivery of maternity care.
- Women are given informed choice in terms of the options available to them during pregnancy, labour and the postnatal period – such as the place of birth, who provides care and where it is given.
- Women have control over the key decisions affecting the content and progress of their care and are supported to have as normal a pregnancy and childbirth experience as possible.
- Women have continuity of care so that they are able to form trusting relationships with those who care for them.

(Extracted from *A Position Statement from the Royal College of Midwives*, available at: **https:// www.rcm.org.uk/position-statements**).

Becoming a parent

The transition towards parenthood is both a social and a psychological process. The changing structure of the family, e.g. the rise of single parenthood, divorce and its meaning, and the inclusion of women in the workforce, the rising age at which women have their first child, all impact on how parenting is experienced by both mothers and fathers. Parenting is affected by wider changes in society such as opportunities for employment and orientation to 'natural' gender roles. The meaning and experience of parenting (e.g. the *autonomous mother*: Bilton et al., 2002) thus change over time and across cultures. This has implications for how parents bring up their children and the results of child-rearing practices. One argument is that the early years are vitally important in the emotional development of children, in which attachment plays an important role. 'Attachment' was once thought to be an aspect of the mother–baby bond but has been criticised for assuming this gender bias. Attachment theory argues that an infant needs to develop a relationship with at least one primary caregiver (male or female) for social and emotional development to occur normally. John Bowlby was an influential figure in the development of this theory (see, for example, Bowlby, 1979).

Activity 8.3   *Reflection*

If you have had a child, think about how your life has changed. What has becoming a parent meant for you and your partner (if you have one)? Think about your lifestyle, your money, your relationship with other family members, your relationship with your partner, your studies.

If you have not had a child of your own, think about how parenthood has impacted on the life of a friend or family member.

As this activity is based on your own experience and observations, there is no outline answer at the end of the chapter.

Attachment in today's Britain may be harder to achieve due to personal aspirations, economic realities and social demands. Sue Gerhardt (2010a) argues that modern child-rearing practices result in acquisitiveness, emotional suppression and a lack of emotional development, emphasising that the early years (0–3 years) are crucial for empathic emotional development. Child-rearing practices are associated with consumerism to produce a *selfish society*. That is to say, parenting takes place within a matrix of other values (the acquisition of cars, houses, holidays) which may conflict with values of sacrifice for child care. Gerhardt suggests that women (and perhaps also men) are being brought back, or take themselves back, into work too early after the child's birth, and a lack of knowledge of emotional development has resulted in a generation of people having a lack of empathic emotional development or connection with others.

Here we see arguments that link social structure and psychological development. It is argued here that capitalism skews values away from human connectivity and an ethic of care based on a relational approach to each other. Child development therefore is a crucial aspect for a healthy society. An implication is that society should invest in 0–3-year-olds to enable them to grow up in safety, love and emotive-relational development. This is expressly discussed in all safeguarding policies (see below) but may not be followed up by the required financing.

Gerhardt's argument is that we should refocus on caring as a real social value and perhaps intro-duce a *caring wage* (2010b), say, £12,000–£16,000 per year at current rates. From this perspective, society has to value care with more than lip service, but in the current economic setting it may be the case that patriarchal and neoliberal (see concept summary box below) capitalist social values are too strong to ensure we do this. Patriarchy devalues women's work, and alongside neoliberal capitalism, does not support child (or elderly) care as paid employment like any other occupation because this is seen as a purely private matter where the cost is to be borne by indi-viduals and families.

Concept summary: Patriarchy

Patriarchy is a social system in which the role of the male as the primary authority figure is central to social organisation, and where fathers hold authority over women, children and property. It implies the institutions of male rule and privilege, and entails female subordi-nation. Many patriarchal societies are also patrilineal, meaning that property and title are inherited by the male lineage.

Neoliberalism is a contemporary form of economic liberalism that emphasises the efficiency of private enterprise, liberalised trade and relatively open markets to promote globalisation. Neoliberals therefore seek to maximise the role of the private sector in determining the political and economic priorities of the world. It involves the redirection of public spending from subsidies (especially what neoliberals call 'indiscriminate subsi-dies') and other spending neoliberals deem wasteful towards broad-based provision of key pro-growth, pro-poor services like primary education, primary healthcare and infra-structure investment.

An example of psychological problems stemming at least in part from social pressures may be the experience of postnatal depression.

Depression: Antenatal and postnatal – some background information

The Clinical Knowledge Summaries (2011) suggest the following.

Depression refers to a spectrum of mental health problems characterised by the absence of positive affect (i.e. a loss of interest and enjoyment in ordinary things and experiences), low mood and a range of associated emotional, cognitive, physical and behavioural symp-toms (National Collaborating Centre for Mental Health, 2004).

Women who are pregnant or postnatal can develop or have the same mental health prob-lems as other adults (National Collaborating Centre for Mental Health, 2007).

The *Diagnostic and Statistical Manual of Mental Disorders* criteria specify that, for depression in the postnatal period, onset is within 4 weeks of birth. However, there is general agreement that onset can occur any time within the first year (SIGN, 2002; Perfetti et al., 2004; Dennis and Hodnett, 2007).

The National Collaborating Centre for Mental Health advises caution in the use of the term 'postnatal depression' as it can be misused to include any mental illness occurring postnatally and may result in other serious illnesses failing to be identified.

Common misconceptions about depression in the postnatal period include:

- Symptoms and effects are less severe than depression at other times.
- It will go away by itself.
- It is entirely due to hormonal changes (National Collaborating Centre for Mental Health, 2007).

Thurtle (1995) argued that the definitions of, and suggestions about, the care of postnatal depression were not agreed across disciplines. There are biological and psychological approaches to understanding this 'illness' which lead to differences regarding the causes of postpartum mental ill health, its treatment or how further research in the area should proceed. Biological and psychological approaches may help to explain depression but they do not present a full picture. What is required is an approach that looks at the stress women experience, suggesting that the conditions in which many women find themselves (such as role conflicts, e.g. mother vs worker), the social expectations placed upon women and support systems, which may or may not be in place, also need to be taken into consideration when trying to understand their experience. Thus postpartum depression may be a rational response to social stressors. This view suggests that the experience is a result of social pressures rather than deficiencies in the biology or psychological make-up of the individual. This argument mirrors a more general discussion around the nature and origin of mental illness – how much of it is organic brain disease, personal psychological difficulties or a result of social situation?

An important finding for Thurtle was that the woman's own perception of postnatal ill health was largely absent from the literature. This means that the experience was being defined by those who may not have experienced it, coming as they may from a 'privileged' position, i.e. not under stress and therefore not having to deal with social pressures. This, of course, raises implications for treatment. Focusing on the individual might lead to drug treatment or individual counselling, whereas what may also be required is changed social circumstances. Nurses who do not understand this process may assist in the treatment of individuals without considering the need to change social policies.

Child development

The Barker theory

So far, we have considered issues around the place of birth and the supervision of birth and suggested there are issues with the woman's experience of childbirth and child care. Conception and pregnancy may seem purely biological events, but even at this time the woman's experiences (including lifestyle) are crucial for healthy babies and for later development of disease in adults.

David Barker (**www.thebarkertheory.org**) suggested that the intrauterine experience was an important factor in the development of heart disease and that this has to be taken into account when considering health services for women. The data, he argues, suggested that low birth weight is related to a greater risk of heart disease. Heart disease is thus not just about adult lifestyle factors or genetics. This 'fetal origins' research suggests that several chronic disorders, which have great implications for public health policy and practice, have their origins in the 9 months before birth. These factors include exposure to toxins in the womb. This then means that environmental health interventions aimed at reducing exposure to the fetus could control several serious public health problems. In June 2011, the Chartered Institute of Environmental Health (CIEH, 2011) set up a task group to review the evidence on the 'fetal origins of health and disease' and ask if this is the beginnings of a major public health advance.

Concept summary: The Barker theory

In coronary heart disease the walls of the arteries supplying blood to the muscle of the heart become hardened, and the channels within them narrowed by deposits of fats. The risk of heart disease is higher in people who were of low birth weight. Risk falls progressively across the range of birth weights. People who weighed 7 lb (3.17 kg) at birth are at lower risk than those who weighed 6 lb (2.72 kg). People who were 9-lb (4.08 kg) babies are at lower risk than those who were 8 lb (3.63 kg). Studies in the USA, in other European countries and in India have confirmed the first observation of the link between heart disease and birth weight, which was made in the UK. It is not babies who were small because they were born prematurely who are at increased risk of later heart disease, but babies who were small because they grew slowly.

Until recently it was thought that the heart was never sacrificed during life in the womb. Like the brain, it is essential for survival and is protected, though there must come a point beyond which protection is no longer possible. In the womb, as the heart pumps blood through the blood vessels in the placenta, the pressures against which it has to work shape the thickness of its muscular walls and the size of its chambers for life. The mother's nutrition shapes the placenta, and the placenta shapes the baby's heart.

(Source: **www.thebarkertheory.org/heart.php**)

What the Barker theory implies is that preconception and the pregnancy itself are crucial periods for later disease development. If society wishes to ensure that the future population is not disadvantaged by the smoking, poor eating and physical exercise activities undertaken by some women, then society may consider intervening in the choices these women make. This is as much a political, social and philosophical question (how much should society intrude?) as a health issue. The question for nurses is: to what degree should the profession intervene in these matters?

Child cognitive development

You will be interacting with and giving care to children of various ages, and will need to understand their physical and psychological development to know what you may reasonably expect a child to be able to understand. You will also need to know the appropriate communication activities you can use. There are other detailed texts on this subject and we refer you to them (for example, Mooney, 2000). The more you work with children, the more you need to acknowledge and understand the following aspects:

- physical growth;
- motor skill development;
- cognitive/intellectual development;
- social/emotional development;
- language development.

One thing to remember is the danger of grouping children and making assumptions based on that grouping. As you have already experienced, no doubt, individual differences occur within similar groupings (for example, across groups of age/ethnicity) as well as across those groupings.

The theorists who have contributed to this understanding include:

- Jean Piaget;
- Lev Vygotsky;
- Erik Erikson;
- John Bowlby;
- John Watson.

Freud also developed a psychosexual theory of human development based on the notion that the sex drive is a basic human motivator. Irvin Yalom argues that what is also important is *death anxiety*, but this becomes more important for adults than children (see Chapter 7). Each theorist illuminates an aspect of child development and this illustrates the varying ways we have of addressing this topic. It is difficult to state with absolute certainty what any child is experiencing in terms of that child's own development or capabilities, but there are broad suggestions that may guide our interaction. As an example, we may consider Piaget's stage theory of cognitive development and Vygotsky's *zone of proximal development.*

For Piaget, children go through four stages (Mooney, 2000).

1. The sensorimotor stage (0–2 years), whereby children experience the world through movement and senses. During this stage children are egocentric, in that they cannot perceive the world from others' viewpoints.
2. The preoperational stage (ages 2–7), whereby children engage in magical thinking and acquiring motor skills. Egocentrism begins strongly and then weakens. Children cannot conserve or use logical thinking.

3. The concrete operational stage (ages 7–11), whereby children begin to think logically but are very concrete in their thinking. Children can now converse and think logically, but only with practical aids. They are no longer egocentric.

4. The formal operational stage (ages 11–16 and onwards), whereby children develop abstract thought and reasoning, and can easily converse and think logically.

This suggests that at each stage the child can think in ways that were not possible in the earlier stages. The stages are discrete.

If this holds, then it has implications for dealing with illness and the way we communicate with children about their health and illness. If abstract thinking does not occur until after 11 years of age, how should children be expected to deal with abstract information about, for example, death or the future progress of conditions such as cystic fibrosis or mental health issues ('mummy's depression', for example)? The critique of this stage theory includes the idea that in reality children are generally more able than Piaget gave them credit for. Their abilities are acquired (more) gradually (or spirally) rather than incrementally, with changes within stages. (Piaget ignored ability differences within stages.) In addition, the emphasis is on what children cannot do; therefore, many findings may have been attributable to the nature of the test he invented. Cognitive development is more dependent on environment and culture than Piaget realised, e.g. training can speed up development. Finally, adults may not be as good at 'formal' or abstract thought as Piaget thought. Despite these revisions and critiques, Piaget's work remains a milestone in understanding.

Vygotsky, in contrast to Piaget, emphasised the social element of cognitive development in that our learning takes place within a social context, with other people, and that this may help to shape and develop our thinking processes (Mooney, 2000). He introduced the idea of 'scaffolding', in which the adult helps the child so that the child can achieve more than s/he could have done alone, and then withdrawing when the child has developed.

This suggests that there is a zone of proximal development, which is the difference between what the child could do on his or her own and with 'able instruction'. This is where learning is most effective. Education, then, should give children experiences that are within their zones of proximal development, thereby encouraging and advancing their individual learning. Children will learn more with adult and peer guidance and instruction within this zone of proximal development. This perspective thus emphasises the need to ensure children get that guidance and instruction, and we may infer that nurses could play this role in helping children to learn about their health and illness alongside parents. It also suggests that children who do not have this input may have impaired cognitive development or may not reach the potential they otherwise would have. Vygotsky's emphasis on collaboration and guidance has potential pitfalls if parents and significant others are too helpful in some cases. An example of that would be an overbearing and controlling parent. It may also be suggested that some children may become lazy and expect help when they can do something on their own.

These two theorists exemplify the complex nature of how children develop, and thus the need for nurses who work with children to reflect carefully on the nature of their interaction and on what assumptions they hold about children. Nurses need to do this with a knowledge drawn from researchers and others. It is also stated often that the parents themselves know their own children better than most, but care is, of course, needed because parents may make assumptions about their children – assumptions which may not be valid.

A good deal of child development literature focuses on what may be considered 'normal' development. The use of the word 'normal' is, of course, open to debate given the complexity of culture, individual capabilities and socialisation practices. To confuse the picture even more, we also need to consider children who have a learning disability. You will have to understand the broad classes of learning disabilities and individualise that knowledge with the children you work with. Some learning disabilities are relatively well known and understood (e.g. Down's syndrome), while others are more difficult for parents to assess or understand (e.g. Asperger's syndrome). To illustrate the point about parents not always knowing best about their own children, the National Autistic Society runs parent courses and training in venues across the UK to help parents understand and deal with their child's experiences.

Autism: Some background

The National Autistic Society website (**www.autism.org.uk**) offers advice and support to parents, carers and other family members. There is an education section and information on communication, therapies and employment. In addition, there is a link to the Autism Act 2009. The Act made two key provisions:

1. that the government produce an adult autism strategy by 1 April 2010;
2. that the Secretary of State for Health issue statutory guidance for local authorities and local health bodies on supporting the needs of adults with autism by 31 December 2010.

The child in society

This section will not address the sociology of the family, as this is done in detail in many other sociology texts (e.g. Bilton et al., 2002). A main point to gather from studies of the family is the cultural variations of what a family is, and how changes in society (for example, the need for a geographically mobile workforce) affect the structure of a family and then, of course, how family life then affects society.

Nurses are called to provide care and organise care for children and the elderly in partnership with family members. Having an understanding of changing family structures (e.g. the growth of single-person households) and values (e.g. towards caring for children and the elderly) illuminates the challenges facing health and social services.

Issues for care are the ageing population and the cost of child care (and thus increasing demands on health services), social understandings of what ageing and childhood mean, and how these affect how we value the care burden of both the elderly and children. That is to say, we have to understand who cares and what it costs.

Nursing is part of the professional paid-care provision, but most care is done by family and friends, often for free or with state support, such as the carer's allowance.

State benefits

There were at least four allowances paid for by the state, which can be found on the website **www.gov.uk** under 'benefits'. The allowances are (2014 rates):

1. Carer's allowance: £61.35 per week, but this will be affected by what is already being received.
2. Attendance allowance: there are two rates: £81.30 and £54.45.
3. Constant attendance allowance: there are four rates, from £132.80 to £33.20.
4. Disability living allowance: the amount you get is down to circumstances and needs.
5. Child benefit allowance: for the eldest or only child, £20.50; for additional children, £13.55 (April 2014 rates), fixed until April 2015.

This is an ever-changing field, and the introduction of universal credit in 2013 supersedes other benefits, including child tax credit. There is also a benefit cap which puts a limit on the total amount of benefit that most people aged 16–64 can get.

The sociology of childhood suggests that there are cultural (and subcultural) variations in the meanings and experiences of childhood. Childhood is not only a biological and psychological stage of development; it has social meaning which changes over time and across cultures. Society in one sense 'defines' (or 'constructs') what childhood is and how we adults relate to children. Note, for example, how the age of sexual consent varies across cultures; note also the differing views on what constitutes child labour both in our time across the world and in history. Chambers (2010) introduces the notion of 'extended' childhood, involving financial support, education and healthcare, which are all products of post-war welfarism. This is manifest in increasing the age for school leavers. For nurses, this now involves concepts of children's rights, including issues around consent. You will address 'Gillick competence' and the Fraser guidelines for consent as part of studies into professional accountability. These reflect changes in views about what children can expect from society.

Activity 8.4   *Team working*

In pairs or threes, discuss what you understand by the word 'child'. When is a child not a child? Think about rights and responsibilities, and how the state defines childhood. Is there a defined end to childhood? If so, who decides and when does it occur?

As the answers to this activity will be based on your own thoughts, there are no answers at the end of the chapter. However, in the answers section you will find a reference to an article discussing this question.

What this means for nurses is the understanding that what is a 'normal' childhood relates to the culture in which that child is brought up. This illustrates the need for cultural competence, i.e. the knowledge of and understanding about cultural practices of those from diverse backgrounds.

How we now experience child care and the meaning of childhood is partly shaped by social conditions. Some of the significant changes over the past three or four decades include the availability of contraception and the termination of unwanted pregnancies. It may be difficult for those under the age of 50 to grasp the importance of the introduction of the control of reproduction for our life choices. For women, the proportion of life devoted to pregnancy and child care has reduced as a consequence of reduced family sizes and contraception, and this has resulted in increased opportunities for employment and education.

'Motherhood' also now includes not just physical care but responsibilities for the psychosocial development of the child, supported and encouraged by the motherhood literature. Motherhood is seen by some as a lifelong identity and a full-time occupation. However, the 'ideal type' of mother is under pressure from structural changes in employment, i.e. female entry into paid work, which entails juggling child care and work. The trend towards *autonomous motherhood* (Bilton et al., 2002, p. 149) is based on the idea that men and women will leave partners when they are unhappy, to have a sex life outside of marriage and to bring up children on their own. This may reflect a positive notion of control or, given the low-wage occupations that many women find themselves in, it can be negative as it results in poverty and hardship. Motherhood and childhood are also shaped by the role of men as fathers and by their own expectations.

Contemporary changes in the economics of employment and the structure of opportunities (i.e. globalisation) for younger age groups may have a profound effect on patterns of family life and childhood. High unemployment rates in Western industrial countries among 16–24-year-olds may impact on their roles and ambitions for family in the future. Some argue that this is already leading to social unrest among this age group (Mason, 2012). Another example of this may be the phenomenon of the so-called 'boomerang generation'. This refers to the frequency with which this generation chooses to live with their parents after a brief period of living on their own – thus boomeranging back to their place of origin. The term can be used to indicate only those members of this age set that actually do return home, not the whole generation. Also, bear in mind that home-leaving practices differ by socioeconomic class, particularly for the middle classes. Parents may have had an expectation of having an 'empty nest', but this is now giving way to the reality of a 'cluttered nest' or 'crowded nest' (see Kathleen Shaputis's book, *The Crowded Nest Syndrome: Surviving the Return of Adult Children*, which takes a critical view of this).

Nurses thus have to understand that fixed notions of motherhood, the family and childhood may not be so fixed after all. The health needs of communities will vary across communities and across cultures. This necessitates suspending our assumptions, based on our own experience, about what 'normal' family life is all about. In the dynamic social conditions in which society now operates, changes can come about very quickly and cannot always be predicted.

A 'sociology of children' (e.g. Prout and Hallett, 2003), which sees the child as social actor, suggests that we should *hear the child's voice* rather than childhood being objectively studied. This is in line with the emphasis on children having a valid status in their own right rather than being the property of parents. This perspective wishes to understand how children engage with society, to explore the worlds they make, and to emphasise their role as active participants, not as merely 'emergent' members of society (with lower status than adults).

Safeguarding children

Other contemporary issues focus around issues of child protection and safety. The adult–child relationship is strained by paedophile fears, which may be akin to a moral panic, resulting in Criminal Records Bureau checks for all who work with children. This imposes a different vision and experience for children in terms of lack of physical exercise and constant adult supervision due to these fears.

The current policy context for children focuses on 'safeguarding'. The UK government defined safeguarding as *[t]he process of protecting children from abuse or neglect, preventing impairment of their health and development, and ensuring they are growing up in circumstances consistent with the provision of safe and effective care that enables children to have optimum life chances and enter adulthood safely* (**www.safeguardingchildren.co.uk**).

Reports are produced to review safeguarding arrangements every 3 years. The first was in 2002. The 2008 report suggests that most children feel safe, but there are some children who were not well served, i.e. those in care homes, children of asylum seekers and those in secure settings. It also notes that access to child protection training, while generally good across agencies, for some staff groups may be limited. This includes nurses and hospital specialists. The Department for Education publishes research reports online: **https://www.gov.uk/government/collections/safeguarding-children**. The Royal College of Nursing (2014) has also produced guidance.

The activities of prominent 'celebrities' such as Jimmy Savile and the resulting findings of Operation Yewtree call into question the nature and extent of child abuse in the UK and challenge our systems and notions around child protection. According to the National Society for the Prevention of Cruelty to Children (NSPCC), there were 1.9 sexual offences per 1,000 children in England and Wales, while in 2013–2014 there were 23,663 recorded sexual offences against children across the whole of the UK (**http://blogs.channel4.com/factcheck/factcheck-paedophiles-britain/18522**). There are methodological issues in surveys and recorded crime which make prevalence data difficult to accept as hard fact. Nonetheless, international surveys suggest a prevalence rate for child abuse of 5–15 per cent for boys and 15–30 per cent of girls. Abuse covers incidents ranging from rape to non-physical abuse. The NSPCC claims that most reported cases of abuse occur in the family (NSPCC, 2014), with associated risk factors of substance misuse, domestic violence, poverty and social exclusion, and mental health difficulties. Children are abused by parents, carers and other family members who live with the child in most reported cases. Clearly, this issue is not going away.

Activity 8.5   *Research and evidence-based practice*

All nurses must have knowledge of these arrangements for child safety and welfare. Access and read the following documents.

Every Child Matters: **https://www.gov.uk/government/uploads/system/uploads/attachment_data/file/272064/5860.pdf**

Department for Children, Schools and Families (2010) *Working Together to Safeguard Children*: **www.education.gov.uk/publications/standard/publicationdetail/page1/DCSF-00305-2010**

Royal College of Nursing (2014) *Safeguarding Children and Young People: Every Nurse's Responsibility*: **http://www.rcn.org.uk/__data/assets/pdf_file/0004/78583/004542.pdf**

You should also be familiar with the main points from the Children Act (2004).

As this activity will draw upon your own responses, there is no outline answer at the end of the chapter.

As for the ill or sick child, there have been developments in what is expected in the care environment itself. See, for example, the National Service Framework for children, young people and maternity services: children in hospital (standard 7: **https://www.gov.uk/government/publications/national-service-framework-children-young-people-and-maternity-services**). This standard states that hospitals must evidence that they give children care centred on their needs, taking in the needs of the family, that children can make informed decisions and that they are consulted when services are planned. There are six themes in the standard which hospitals need to address and could form the basis for evaluating the standards of care offered to children. For example, theme 5 is around *safety and good quality care*, which includes, among a list of things, *provision for parents to stay overnight, access to meals for parents and space for relaxation.*

Nurses with responsibility for checking standards of the quality of care will need to address these standards in their own workplaces. That means all nurses. This will require management and leadership skills.

Chapter summary

- Care provision for pregnant women and for children may be subject to particular views about who knows what is best for client groups, resulting in arguments about who is best placed to decide what care should be and how it should be delivered.
- At the heart of many approaches are the values placed on particular activities. It is important to try to understand how those values come to be and to challenge our own assumptions.

continued . . . •••

- The stages of child development are complex, and have been the subject of much study.
- Family life in modern Britain is varied and the experience of parenthood is open to both psychological and social pressures.
- Many people are dealing with complex demands made upon them, which then shape how their children grow up and the sort of society they experience.

Activities: brief outline answers

Activity 8.2 Research and evidence-based practice

Exploring the United Nations Millennium Development Goals website will have enabled you to find out that 350,000 women a year die from complications during childbirth, and that 99 per cent of these are in the developing world. More than a million children per year are left motherless as a result.

Activity 8.4 Team working

When is a child not a child? See Joan Smith's (2010) article of that name in *The Independent*: **www.independent.co.uk/opinion/commentators/joan-smith/joan-smith-when-is-a-child-not-a-child-1982689.html**.

Further reading

Bilton, A, Bonnett, K, Jones, P, Lawson, T, Skinner, D, Stanworth, M and Webster, A (2002) *Introductory Sociology*, 4th edn. Basingstoke: Palgrave Macmillan, pp. 238–239.

For further reading on the medicalisation of motherhood and reproductive technologies.

Chenery-Morris, S and McLean, M (2012) *Normal Midwifery Practice.* London: Sage/Learning Matters.

A good, reader-friendly introduction to maternity care.

Kent, J (2000) *Social Perspectives on Pregnancy and Childbirth for Midwives, Nurses and the Caring Professions.* Maidenhead: Open University Press.

Raynor, M and England, C (2010) *Psychology for Midwives: Pregnancy, Childbirth and Puerperium.* Maidenhead: Open University Press.

Wyness, M (2006) *Childhood and Society: An Introduction to the Sociology of Childhood.* Basingstoke: Palgrave Macmillan.

Three accessible textbooks giving sociological and psychological perspectives on maternity and child care.

Useful websites

www.nice.org.uk

The website of the National Institute for Health and Care Excellence.

www.nct.org.uk

The website of the National Childbirth Trust.

www.rcm.org.uk

The Royal College of Midwives is the midwifery equivalent of the Royal College of Nursing.

www.rcog.org.uk

The Royal College of Obstetricians and Gynaecologists – another useful source of information.

https://www.gov.uk/childrens-services/safeguarding-children

The government's website, hosting a plethora of guidance, reports and research.

Chapter 9
Mental health and learning disabilities

> ### NMC Standards for Pre-registration Nursing Education
>
> This chapter will address the following competencies:
>
> **Domain 1: Professional values**
> **Mental health nurses** must work with people of all ages using values-based mental health frameworks. They must use different methods of engaging people, and work in a way that promotes positive relationships focused on social inclusion, human rights and recovery, that is, a person's ability to live a self-directed life, with or without symptoms, that they believe is meaningful and satisfying.
>
> 4. All nurses must work in partnership with service users, carers, families, groups, communities and organisations. They must manage risk, and promote health and wellbeing while aiming to empower choices that promote self-care and safety.
>
> **Learning disabilities nurses** must promote the individuality, independence, rights, choice and social inclusion of people with learning disabilities and highlight their strengths and abilities at all times while encouraging others do the same. They must facilitate the active participation of families and carers.
>
> **Domain 2: Communication**
> **Mental health nurses** must practise in a way that focuses on the therapeutic use of self. They must draw on a range of methods of engaging with people of all ages experiencing mental health problems, and those important to them, to develop and maintain therapeutic relationships. They must work alongside people, using a range of interpersonal approaches and skills to help them explore and make sense of their experiences in a way that promotes recovery.
>
> **Learning disabilities nurses** must use complex communication and interpersonal skills and strategies to work with people of all ages who have learning disabilities and help them to express themselves. They must also be able to communicate and negotiate effectively with other professionals, services and agencies, and ensure that people with learning disabilities, their families and carers, are fully involved in decision-making.
>
> **Domain 3: Nursing practice and decision-making**
> **Mental health nurses** must draw on a range of evidence-based psychological, psycho-social and other complex therapeutic skills and interventions to provide person-centred support and care across all ages, in a way that supports self-determination and aids recovery.

They must also promote improvements in physical and mental health and wellbeing and provide direct care to meet both the essential and complex physical and mental health needs of people with mental health problems.

Learning disabilities nurses must have an enhanced knowledge of the health and developmental needs of all people with learning disabilities, and the factors that might influence them. They must aim to improve and maintain their health and independence through skilled direct and indirect nursing care. They must also be able to provide direct care to meet the essential and complex physical and mental health needs of people with learning disabilities.

Domain 4: Leadership, management and team working
Mental health nurses must contribute to the leadership, management and design of mental health services. They must work with service users, carers, other professionals and agencies to shape future services, aid recovery and challenge discrimination and inequality.

Learning disabilities nurses must exercise collaborative management, delegation and supervision skills to create, manage and support therapeutic environments for people with learning disabilities.

Chapter aims

By the end of this chapter you will be able to:

- consider how mental health and illness are variously experienced and defined;
- relate physical and mental illness together;
- discuss the values-based approach to learning disabilities care;
- suggest why care in some cases can be abusive or of poor quality.

Introduction

In this chapter we will explore some psychosocial issues in the fields of mental health and learning disability nursing, which will be useful to all nurses who will need to have a broad understanding of any person who might come into their care, irrespective of their field of practice. We will discuss the different ways of understanding mental health/illness ('madness') which challenge our understanding of what is normal behaviour. Does madness arise in the individual or is society mad itself? Is 'madness' therefore a rational reaction to some very irrational social situations? Mental illness, of course, is not just a function of how society works; there are very real experiences that cause distress for people.

We will also look at the psychological and social issues that impact on the care of those with learning disabilities. An important issue is the social provision of care for people with learning disabilities linked to their perceived status as full citizens.

Mental health

Nurses are placed in clinical settings which will vary in their understanding and experience of mental illness and will work with health professionals who have also potentially different ideas about what mental health and illness are. Therefore, it is necessary to be aware of the differences and explore the evidence for certain assessments, diagnosis and treatment options.

So, the question about what mental illness is may not be as easy to answer as we may at first think. There are various ways of thinking about 'madness', ranging from orthodox psychiatry using the *Diagnostic and Statistical Manual IV* and now 5 (DSM-IV and DSM-5: American Psychiatric Association, 2000, 2013) or the *International Classification of Disease Manual* (World Health Organization, 2015), through to the 'myth of mental illness' position of some radical psychiatrists, e.g. Thomas Szasz. The postnatal depression (PND) discussion in Chapter 8 illustrates the multidimensional nature of some experiences.

Activity 9.1   *Reflection*

What do you understand by these terms?

- mental health;
- mental illness;
- madness.

As this activity is based on your own reflection, there are no answers at the end of the chapter; however, you may compare your answers with the discussion below.

What is considered as 'madness' is problematic in a very subtle way. We have to consider what we mean by *normality* if we are going to define madness as a deviation from the norm. Many 'normal' people have beliefs which are similar to those labelled as mad. In the context of a religious ceremony, hearing God's voice may be seen as perfectly normal; elsewhere it may be seen as evidence of psychosis.

There are at least two ways of thinking about this: individual or social. The first is that mental illness is what the medics say it is. The focus here is on the individual: sanity or insanity arises from within the individual as an organic brain disease or disordered thinking. The individual must be medically examined, or psychoanalysed, and treated with surgery, medications or some form of talking therapy, such as cognitive behavioural therapy. PND in this view arises from within the individual and antidepressants may be the way to treat it. However, even this 'madness lies within the individual' view is not straightforward.

Darian Leader in *What Is Madness?* (Leader, 2011) illustrates the different professional approaches to understanding 'madness'. One idea he discusses is how professionals, psychiatrists on the one hand and psychoanalysts on the other, see a difference between *symptom* and *structure*. A symptom is what the client says he or she is experiencing. For example, he argues that current psychiatry accepts the diagnostic category of social phobia as being the same thing as the symptoms outlined in DSM-IV. Thus, the psychiatrist takes a list of symptoms and then compares that to the diagnosis in DSM.

The symptoms of social phobia include excessive shyness, self-consciousness and anxiety in everyday social situations, blushing and shortness of breath. If a client tells the psychiatrist that s/he has these symptoms, then social phobia can be diagnosed. The DSM will list these symptoms. Treatment may then focus on control of these symptoms through the use of certain medications.

Leader argues, however, that we need a different, psychoanalytical, approach to engage in careful dialogue with the client to uncover the underlying *structure* and not just outline the symptoms. What does he mean by this?

If a person complains of shyness, blushing and sweating (symptoms), this may be because s/he thinks s/he will say the wrong things and lose face in a social setting. This is a 'neurotic structure' exposed through discourse with the person. Another person with the same surface symptoms may do so because s/he believes, or knows, that other people can read his or her thoughts, a 'psychotic structure' again revealed through dialogue. Two deep structures exist, one based on a questioning of one's value to another (am I lovable?); the other is based on a delusional certainty that one's thoughts can be read. There are two different *structures* but with the same surface *symptoms*. Therefore, diagnosing social phobia based on the DSM list of symptoms will miss the difference between a person's neurotic mental structure and psychotic mental structure.

> ### The Diagnostic and Statistical Manual of Mental Disorders (DSM-5)
>
> DSM-5 is a manual published by the American Psychiatric Association that includes all currently recognised mental health disorders. An example in the DSM is *social anxiety disorder*, which is also known as social phobia. This is an anxiety disorder characterised by intense fear in social situations, causing considerable distress and impaired ability to function in at least some parts of daily life.

Social madness

This is a second way of understanding illness. If society does not actually *cause* illness, then the way society is organised may itself be 'mad'. Thurtle's (1995) view on the social expectations placed on women, as causative factors in PND, exemplifies this approach. This focus, from the individual to society, is clearly outlined by Eric Fromm (Goodman, 2014).

Eric Fromm (1900–1980) based his work (2002, first published 1956) on a notion that humans have an essential nature. He wished to analyse the *pathology of society* which would prevent humans from developing this essential nature to its full potential. His analysis suggested that, for example, the development and deployment of nuclear weapons and the dumbing down of civil society through mass-media 'entertainments' show evidence of social pathology. In contemporary society the elevation of 'the markets' as the last arbiters of economic life, which then demand austerity measures, regardless of the social consequences, is also evidence of an insane society.

Fromm gave a definition of mental health:

> *Mental health is characterised by the ability to love and create, by the emergence from incestuous ties to clan and soil, by a sense of identity based on one's experience of self as the subject and agent of one's powers, by the grasp of reality inside and outside of ourselves, that is, by the development of objectivity and reason.*
> (Fromm, 2002, p. 67)

His was an attempt to state what mental health is, to give us a yardstick by which we could measure how well, or badly, societies promote health. His analysis of capitalism was that this form of social organisation was itself insane.

Our ability to *develop* mental health has a basis in individual factors, so an organic brain disease such as a tumour obviously inhibits health, to say the least. However, *mental health is mostly about what society makes possible.* Thus, this is *not* about adjusting the individual to norms of society, an approach taken by mainstream psychiatry and clinical psychology. The adjustment of the individual to society happens in the treatment of PND. Society places often unachievable role expectations upon women and then 'adjusts' them through the use of drugs, or counselling, to these social conditions. Faced with a care burden and social isolation and the need to be the ideal 'mother', many women break down. The 'madness in the individual' answer is to adjust that woman to her conditions. A 'social madness' perspective may suggest that we organise social expectations and conditions differently so that women are not socially isolated, and have more realistic expectations placed upon them.

Health, for Fromm, *must be defined in terms of the adjustment of society to the needs of man* (2002, p. 70), and not the other way around. So, to address PND, the social structures within which women find themselves and the role expectations that society places upon them ought to be 'adjusted'. It could then be suggested that nurses who work to administer medications, or who provide counselling, merely perpetuate the insane social system rather than challenging it. Nurses themselves may have internalised 'ideal types' of motherhood and uncritically accepted the current social organisation of childbirth, child rearing and motherhood. They may ironically often fall prey themselves to the same social processes and take medications to adjust themselves to the needs of the family and employment.

Fromm's perspective of the social nature of insanity may be seen operating also within the Critical Psychiatry Network (see below).

Activity 9.2	*Critical thinking*

Female genital mutilation/female circumcision is seen by most Westerners as an abusive social practice. Any society that sees this as acceptable is open to be interpreted as an example of Fromm's insane society.

Consider Western 'normal' social practices. Discuss what could be seen as evidence of insanity, even though we do not think it is. For example, in recent history the incarceration of people with mental illnesses in asylums was seen as 'normal' practice, but from today's perspective it may appear, if not abusive, then certainly far from satisfactory. Consider aspects of the care of those with learning disabilities or of the institutionalisation of older people.

An outline answer to this activity is given at the end of the chapter.

Critical Psychiatry Network

The Critical Psychiatry Network first met in 1999 to discuss compulsory treatment in the community and reviewable detention, and to oppose these developments. To understand critical psychiatry we must consider the recent context in which medicine and psychiatry have been practised, which we allude to above. The following argument is a perspective from critical psychiatry.

We have already noted criticism of the medical profession, and the idea of the medicalisation of everyday life, e.g. a pill for every 'ill', even if the illness is not illness at all but a problem with life. This is in addition to the public's disaffection with the medical profession. We have already noted that the assumption that science and technology can answer society's most complex problems has been thrown open to doubt. As medicine has become more influenced by technology and science, it has lost contact with basic human values of respect for the individual's beliefs and preferences. The situation in psychiatry is that neuroscience, based on distorted media coverage of high-profile 'failures' of community care in which those with mental illness have been freed to kill, has driven a political agenda in which risk reduction is of paramount importance. We now have laws forcing people to take medication. There has always been a split within psychiatry between care and healing on the one hand, and coercion and social control on the other. The law now supports coercion over care.

There are three elements to critical psychiatry. It challenges the dominance of clinical neuroscience in psychiatry but does not exclude it; it introduces a strong ethical perspective on psychiatric knowledge and practice; it politicises mental health issues.

Critical psychiatry is deeply sceptical about the claims of neuroscience to explain psychosis and other forms of emotional distress by locating illness only within the individual. The claims of the pharmaceutical industry for the role of psychotropic drugs in the 'treatment' of psychiatric conditions are questioned perhaps as self-serving and far too narrow an approach. Drugs may have a role, but not as the first 'go to' treatment for illness. More importance needs to be given to dealing with social factors, such as unemployment, bad housing, poverty, stigma and social isolation.

Those who use mental health services may regard these factors as more important than drugs. The medical model in psychiatry is rejected in favour of a social model. This is even more important in a multicultural society characterised by deep inequalities.

Critical psychiatry therefore brings a political perspective to mental health issues. The biomedical (neuroscientific) model locates distress in the disordered function of the individual's mind/brain, individualising and relegating social issues to a secondary role. This is problematic because it completely overlooks the role of poverty and social exclusion in psychosis. Within this view the relationship between medic and patient is redefined in that, although psychiatrists are experts by profession, service users are experts by experience. The best outcomes will only be achieved when these two types of expertise can work together.

The implication for nursing is that, without this critique, nursing practice may become merely a cog in the bigger machine of an apolitical and asocial psychiatric practice. This perspective therefore calls for a social policy and political role for nursing practice rather than just trying to adapt the individual to poor social conditions through the use of talking therapies and medications.

Mental illness therefore has a social dimension to it, and here we see how society and individual psychology work together in creating a person's experience. We have not emphasised the biological and genetic preconditions for mental illness because we are concentrating on the social and psychological aspects. Clearly, the experience of 'madness' for people is very real and is not only the creation of social 'forces'.

Illness as a crisis

If issues such as social exclusion, stigma, bad housing and consumerism add to psychological suffering, we may more fully understand the real suffering individuals endure. This suffering may then be exacerbated when the illness acts as a 'crisis'. We have already noted the stress response and the development of adaptive or maladaptive coping mechanisms. We may then note that our normal coping strategies may not work when confronted with new experiences, for example, within a psychotic episode. A crisis happens when our various coping strategies do not work and a state of despair and disorganisation results. Many of us will find a way out of crisis; in other words, the crisis is self-limiting, but if we are not able to resolve it then help may be needed.

Crisis theory

Here we are concerned with how people deal with a crisis and how they psychologically adapt as a result. We assume that our psyche tries to balance itself, similarly to physiological homeostasis. If we are knocked off balance we experience disequilibrium and this results in the questioning of, and changes with, our self and social identity. The birth of a child, for some, is a crisis. We move from one identity to another and this may bring up feelings of uncertainty. PND may then result.

Moos and Schaefer (1984) suggest the following changes can occur as a result of a physical illness. We will apply this structure to understand PND (note: we are not defining childbirth as a physical illness).

- Identity: e.g. the woman changes her identity from being single, a career woman or a partner/wife to being a mother.
- Location: e.g. the woman may have had to cope with being in hospital, with strangers and in institutional care. Then, upon discharge home, she may have to face restrictions in her own home due to loss of freedom and mobility due to the baby's all-encompassing needs.
- Role: e.g. from an active independent person to non-active, passive recipient. The woman could perceive herself to be out of control or as becoming a 'victim'.
- Social support: childbirth may result in isolation and enforced social withdrawal. There may be a loss of social contact of friends and family after the initial period of celebration. Or a new baby, being the centre of attention, brings overbearing social support and often unsaid, but nonetheless real, social expectations such as bonding or attachment, backed by theorists such as John Bowlby, or the expectation that the new mum expresses the 'maternal instinct', which in fact the woman may not have.
- Future: the future may be uncertain; the woman may not be able to make plans, or may have to cancel plans. Her responsibilities are all uncertain.

Physical illness and psychological sequelae

Moos and Schaefer apply this structure to the understanding of physical illness. In addition to the changes to self-identity and social identity, the problems of physical illness may be exacerbated by the disease itself, in that there may be elements of unpredictability. The illness may have been unexpected and so an individual's coping strategies have not been developed. The information about the illness may be unclear or ambiguous. On the basis of the illness, quick, life-changing decisions may have to be made. The outcome is unclear and questions about prognosis and death may be unresolved. The person may well have very limited or no previous experience.

In these ways physical illness has 'psychological sequelae' (Latin *sequela*: 'that which follows'), that is to say, physical illness may be followed by psychological issues for the patient. An example is posttraumatic stress disorder following injury on the battlefield or our example of PND following childbirth. Nurses involved in the physical care of adults will base their care planning and assessment on various models (e.g. Roper et al., 2000), which may address the psychosocial sequelae to varying degrees. Or they may not.

Activity 9.3   *Critical thinking*

Using Moos and Schaefer's crisis theory above, choose a physical illness and think through the possible steps that a person may go through to end up in psychological crisis.

An outline answer to this activity is given at the end of the chapter.

To explore this link further we will examine a common experience: depression.

Depression

House (2003) argues that *feeling unhappy* about being ill is understandable. However, he argues it is the case that the majority of people do *not* suffer from sustained low mood when they have a physical disease, even a chronic and disabling one. For those who *do* have a depressive disorder alongside a physical illness, the result seems to be a lower quality of life, and worse outcomes from treatment. The recognition and treatment of co-existent depression ought therefore to be a part of the management of all chronic disease.

Lustman and Anderson (2002) argue that patients with diabetes are twice as likely to experience depression as those without diabetes. The odds of depression are similar in type 1 and type 2 diabetes and are significantly higher in women than in men. Moreover, the psychiatric condition presents as major depression or elevated depression symptoms in 11 per cent and 31 per cent, respectively, of adults with diabetes. The course of depression in diabetes tends to be severe, with recurrences being the norm and not the exception. Following successful treatment, fewer than 10 per cent of patients remain depression-free over the ensuing five years, and afflicted patients tend to suffer about one episode of major depression annually. Depression has additional importance in diabetes because of its association with poor compliance with diabetes treatment.

Gill and Hatcher (2003) undertook a Cochrane review to determine whether antidepressants are clinically effective for those experiencing depression following physical illness. They argue that depression in the physically unwell is common and an important cause of morbidity. There are problems with diagnosing depression in the physically ill, which may lead to under-recognition and under-treatment. The depression frequently has a poor outcome, and patients often have an increased morbidity and mortality – that is to say, the depressed suffer more illness and death. Depressed physically ill patients have more investigations and treatments than the non-depressed; they have worse functions, and are also less likely to comply with treatment.

The National Institute for Health and Care Excellence (NICE) guideline for depression (**www. nice.org.uk/CG90**) suggests screening should be undertaken in primary care and general hospital settings for depression in high-risk groups – for example, those with a past history of depression, significant physical illnesses causing disability or other mental health problems, such as dementia. Healthcare professionals should bear in mind the potential physical causes of depression and the possibility that depression may be caused by medication, and consider screening if appropriate. Screening for depression should include the use of at least two questions concerning mood and interest, such as: 'During the last month, have you often been bothered by feeling down, depressed or hopeless?' and 'During the last month, have you often been bothered by having little interest or pleasure in doing things?'

Nurses need to be aware of the psychological consequences of physical illness, so that they can:

- respond to distress, as appropriate;
- refer when appropriate;
- be aware of distress as a cause of health behaviour.

Other issues

So far, we have examined the varying definitions of and approaches to mental illness and briefly examined the multifactorial nature of the experience. We have suggested that physical illness has psychological consequences and this works also in reverse.

Other common issues you will need to explore in more depth include:

1. substance abuse;
2. suicide – risk assessment and referral;
3. the range of disorders and their aetiologies;
4. support services in primary care and in hospital. Activity 9.4 will help you begin to address this.

The further reading and useful websites at the end of this chapter will also help you on these topics.

Finally, there is an issue of 'parity of esteem' between mental and physical health, and a strain upon the provision and resourcing for mental illness. Nick Clegg, when deputy Prime Minister, stated that it was *just plain wrong* to treat mental health services as the poor cousin of physical health in the NHS, citing too much *ignorance, prejudice and discrimination* (BBC, 2014a). Issues arising for people included:

• Over 50 per cent stated stigma and discrimination were as bad as, or worse than, the illness itself.
• Over 25 per cent waited over a year to tell their family about their illness.
• Nearly 25 per cent of young people said stigma stopped them going to school.

The UK government launched a strategy for mental health in 2014 (Department of Health, 2014). It stated:

> *People who use mental health services, and those that care for them, continue to report gaps in provision and long waits for services. There is still insufficient support within communities for people with mental health problems. In some areas there have been stories of people of all ages being transferred sometimes hundreds of miles to access a bed. We are not yet making an impact on the enormous gap in physical health outcomes for those with mental health problems.*
> (Department of Health, 2014, p. 5)

The strategy sets out 25 recommendations to address these and other issues. There is clearly some work to be done. Criticisms of mental health provision emerged from the Royal College of Nursing, who stated that staff cuts and bed shortages were leaving mental health services under *unprecedented strain* (BBC, 2014b). A clinician writes: *I love working in mental health – but I can't do a good job on a shoestring* (*The Guardian*, 2014). Bear in mind that both statements are written from certain points of view; nonetheless, they strike a chord with the tone of other reports around mental health care provision, such as that of the charity YoungMinds. Doward (2014) cites Sarah Brennan, chief executive officer of YoungMinds: *For all the welcome policy announcements from government about children and young people's mental health, the picture on the ground for many children, young people and their families is of services in crisis.*

The President of the Royal College of Psychiatrists was reported (Boseley, 2014) to have said: *Less than a third of people with common mental health problems get any treatment at all – a situation the nation would not tolerate if they had cancer.* If this is true, it illustrates just how far 'parity of esteem' has to travel.

Activity 9.4   *Research and evidence-based practice*

You will need to understand the role and function of the community psychiatric nurse and the hospital psychiatric liaison nurse. When it is appropriate (and in negotiation with your clinical mentor), in your next clinical placement try to spend some time with nurses in these roles, and ask them about how they see mental illness and the various treatment options open to them.

As the answer to this activity will depend on your own situation and experience, no outline answer is given at the end of the chapter.

Learning disabilities: a values-based approach to care

You may have concluded that much of the previous discussion regarding children and mental health issues will also apply to people with a learning disability. There are, of course, the same ambiguities in some cases of diagnosis and treatment, and of the role for carers and challenges for society in providing that care.

The British Institute for Learning Disabilities (BILD) has a vision for learning disabilities care in society which sets out the sorts of values that should underpin how we approach the care of people with a learning disability. The organisation states that its vision is one where society treats those with a learning disability as equal citizens, with the right support to enable them to live their lives as they want to, rather than having to accept what is merely available or on offer. The focus here is on advocacy, human rights, positive behaviour support and developing a workforce that provides that support. You may see this vision statement as self-evident, but an examination of the history of learning disabilities care in the UK demonstrates why these values have to be clearly expressed.

Activity 9.5   *Research and evidence-based practice*

How were people with a learning disability cared for from 1900 up to the 1980s? What values underpinned that care approach?

Go to the Learning Disability History research group, based at the Open University (**www. open.ac.uk/hsc/ldsite/research_grp.html**), where you will find publications on this topic. See particularly Welshman and Walmsley (2006).

An outline answer to this activity is given at the end of the chapter.

Despite changes in care philosophy, people with a learning disability have suffered neglect, abuse and poor-quality care. This suggests that their needs are not always properly understood, assessed or catered for. The *Joint Investigation into the Provision of Services for People with Learning Disabilities at Cornwall Partnership NHS Trust* stated:

> *some individuals, as the Trust has acknowledged, have suffered abuse including physical, emotional and environmental abuse . . . some people using its services have had to endure years of abusive practices and some have suffered real injury as a result.*

> *Institutional abuse was widespread, preventing people from exercising their rights to independence, choice and inclusion. One person spent 16 hours a day tied to their bed or wheelchair, for what staff wrongly believed was for that person's own protection.*

> (Healthcare Commission and CSCI, 2006, p. 8)

Since that serious report we have had the case of Sutton and Merton Primary Care Trust in which, for example:

> *[t]he model of care was based on the convenience of the service providers rather than the needs of individuals. For example during meal times some people's shoulders were wrapped in a large sheet of blue tissue paper, and they were then fed at a speed that would not allow for any enjoyment of the food.*
> (Healthcare Commission, 2007, p. 3)

Following that, we have had the Winterbourne View case in Bristol (see Chapter 2) and allegations of abuse by staff at a day centre in Penzance (BBC, 2011d). We must state again that we are not arguing that all care is abusive. Rather, it is to illustrate again how values become institutionalised, internalised, common and not open to internal critique. This also illuminates why organisations such as BILD highlight the values-based nature of learning disability work and why there needs to be consistent monitoring both externally and internally of the care services we offer.

Activity 9.6 — *Critical thinking and reflection*

- Look up the summary of the *Joint Investigation into the Provision of Services* report at: **www. cqc.org.uk**.
- Why do you think this might have happened?
- What were the safeguards to prevent such things happening?
- What does this case say about the way the clients were valued as human beings?
- What causes people to behave in an abusive way? Burnout? Detachment? Group think? Peer pressure?
- What can we as practitioners do to ensure we don't fall into the same pernicious behaviour patterns?

An outline answer to this activity is given at the end of the chapter.

The policy documents outlined in the executive summary of that report (Healthcare Commission and CSCI, 2006) lay the foundations for our approach to care and should be available to, and understood by, all nurses who are responsible for care provision. They include the *Valuing People* report (Department of Health, 2001c) and the *No Secrets* guidance (Department of Health, 2000). Other important legislation includes the Human Rights Act 1998, the Disability Discrimination Act 1995, the Mental Capacity Act 2005 and the Equality Act 2010. You must be aware of the provisions of that legislation and apply it in clinical practice.

Seeking Consent: Working with People with LD (Department of Health, 2001a) focuses on the appropriate procedures for seeking consent from those with the capacity to give it. It discusses the concept of *capacity* and includes brief examples, illustrating typical scenarios. It also details the type of information people are likely to need in order to make an informed-consent decision. Part two looks at what should be done when adults are unable to give or refuse consent. It explains the use of *advance directives* and how a person's *best interests* can be determined. The third section covers consent to involvement in therapeutic and non-therapeutic research. The final section deals with decisions connected to withdrawing or withholding life-prolonging treatment.

Healthcare for All (Michael, 2008) argued that, despite the Discrimination Disability Act and the Mental Capacity Act 2005, people with learning disabilities have higher levels of unmet need and receive less effective treatment. Among the reasons given was that not enough attention (by health services) is given to making reasonable adjustments to support the delivery of equal treatment. These adjustments should take into account communication difficulties. Parents and carers often found their opinions and assessment ignored by professionals and they struggled to be effective partners in care. This report also points out that health service staff, particularly those working in general healthcare, have very limited knowledge about learning disability. They are also unfamiliar with the legislative framework and commonly fail to understand that a right to equal treatment does not mean treatment should be the same. In addition, the health needs of those with a learning disability are poorly understood.

This report outlines eight reasons for the issues raised, one of which was that compliance with the law (e.g. Disability Discrimination and Mental Capacity) is not effectively monitored. There is also poor performance management in primary, community, secondary and specialist care services. Another aspect was that training and education about learning disability in the NHS is very limited. This results in ignorance and fear, which reinforces negative attitudes and values, and then failure to treat people with dignity and respect.

In 2010 the Department of Health published *Valuing People Now*, a new 3-year strategy for people with learning disabilities. *Valuing People Now* responded to the main recommendations in *Healthcare for All* (Michael, 2008). In 2009 the Parliamentary and Health Ombudsman Report, *Six Lives: The Provision of Public Services to People with Learning Disabilities*, catalogued six distressing cases of abusive care and revealed the following:

- There were significant and distressing failures in service across health and social care.
- One person died as a consequence of public service failure. It is likely the death of another individual could have been avoided, if the care and treatment provided had not fallen so far below the relevant standards.

- People with learning disabilities experienced prolonged suffering and poor care, and some of these failures were for disability-related reasons.
- Some public bodies failed to live up to human rights principles, especially those of dignity and equality.
- Many organisations responded inadequately to the complaints made against them, which left family members feeling drained and demoralised.

Although based on only six cases, these cannot be dismissed as isolated incidents, given the growing evidence of poor care across care services.

In 2014, a report *Winterbourne View: Time for Change* (Transforming Care and Commissioning Steering Group, 2014) focused on inappropriate institutionalised care following a government pledge to move people from inappropriate care into community care locations. It argues that pledge has not been fulfilled; in fact, more people are being admitted than discharged. There are several recommendations in the report, starting with urgently closing inappropriate inpatient institutions and drawing up a charter of rights.

Therefore, following the history of institutionalised and deindividualised care for learning disabilities, and alongside a raft of policy statements and legislation concerning human rights and values-based approaches to care, it appears to be the case that some people with learning disabilities continue to receive less than optimum care. We have already hinted at why this may be the case. The social devaluing of groups of people may be one mechanism for fostering uncaring and devaluing actions. Social role valorisation (SRV) recognises this process.

Social role valorisation theory

SRV is concerned with creating or supporting socially valued roles for people on the basis that if people hold a valued social role they are more likely to receive status, acceptance and the services they need. Consider the valued social role of a doctor, for example. The 'good things' in life include dignity, respect, acceptance, education and belonging. Wolf Wolfensberger (1992), who formulated this theory, defined SRV as: the application of what science can tell us about the enablement, establishment, enhancement, maintenance, and/or defence of valued social roles for people (Wolfensberger, 1995).

SRV is relevant to two groups of people in society: those who are already socially devalued (those with learning disabilities) and those who are at heightened risk of becoming devalued. SRV is then a response to the social devaluation of groups of people. Enhancing the perceived value of the social roles of a person or class is called SRV, and doing so is role valorising. There are two major broad strategies for pursuing this goal for (devalued) people:

1. enhancement of people's social image in the eyes of others;
2. enhancement of their competences, in the widest sense of the term.

In applying this to those with learning disabilities, nurses could adopt these two strategies in their attempts to revalue a devalued group so that they can enjoy the 'good things' society bestows upon its valued members (**www.socialrolevalorization.com/index.html**).

The Royal College of Nursing guide (2011)

Finally, in 2011, the Royal College of Nursing published guidance for nursing staff in *Meeting the Health Needs of People with Learning Disabilities* (Royal College of Nursing, 2011a). The 2011 guide arose from work done in 2006 in response to calls for those with a learning disability to have equitable access and treatment. This is a very useful guide which outlines key policy statements and practical issues around physical care and knowledge about certain conditions. This report implicitly accepts the findings of the *Healthcare for All* report (Michael, 2008) – specifically, the issue around education of healthcare staff.

One way staff may address the needs of those with learning disabilities is the *patient passport system* (Kent, 2008). The passport contains information on the patient's individual needs to help in the care-planning process. This also allows the patient to be part of the decision-making process.

Activity 9.7   *Critical thinking and team working*

Go to the Healthcare Commission and CSCI (2006) report, mentioned above, and read page 8. Access the reports mentioned and discuss the main values and positions taken by those reports.

An outline answer to this activity is given at the end of the chapter.

Chapter summary

- There are important differences in the way that professionals think about what mental illness is and the causes for 'abnormal' behaviour. This has implications for treatment and the nurse's role.
- Care provision may be subject to particular views about who knows what is best for client groups, which result in argument about who is best placed to decide what care should be and how it should be delivered.
- The history of institutional care illustrates how society valued and understood those with learning disabilities and mental illness. The current practice issues (of abusive and poor-quality care) also illustrate the vulnerability of clients and reflect certain social practices and attitudes towards them.
- At the heart of many approaches is the values people place on certain activities and we must understand how those values come to be and challenge our own assumptions in this regard.

Activities: brief outline answers

Activity 9.2 Critical thinking

According to Reuters news agency, the USA spent $1 trillion on the war in Afghanistan (**www.reuters.com**: 14 January 2010). According to the BBC (**http://news. bbc.co.uk**: 22 September 2010), the Trident nuclear missile system may cost between £15 billion and £35 billion to replace. Set these figures against the fact that 80 per cent of humanity live on less than $10 a day (**www.globalissues.org/article/26/poverty- facts-and-stats#src1**).

Activity 9.3 Critical thinking

Moos and Schaefer's crisis theory could, for example, be applied to the case of a 58-year-old man newly diagnosed with type 2 diabetes.

- Identity: a shift from an identity of healthy 'macho' 'eat and drink what I like' virility to one of a slightly feminised concern with diet. This illness challenges male identity as being strong and in control.
- Location: although diabetes does not make a person house-bound, he has to consider activity levels and monitoring of blood glucose and the location of equipment to do so. For example, he might need to think like this: 'What if I go down the pub and feel tired – do I have what I need?'
- Role: e.g. from an active independent person to being 'active with care as to my blood sugars' and a passive recipient of observation and control. The man could perceive himself to be out of control or become a 'victim' as he has to cede control to health professionals.
- Social support: will his workmates understand his new regime regarding diet and alcohol? Does his wife support the new regimes he has to go through? 'Does anyone know in my family what it feels like to have diabetes and the reasons for monitoring and medications?'
- Future: 'Will I lose my eyesight? Will I get circulation problems? Will this affect how I look to my wife? The future now is all about the monitoring and treatment of the diabetes to prevent severe complications. Gone are the free-and-easy days when I did not think about my health at all; gone are the days when I could eat and drink what I liked, when I liked and how much I liked.'
- He might assume the identity of 'diabetic' and limit what he does unnecessarily through misunderstanding of the nature if the illness. He has lost his identity as a strong independent man and assumed the mantle of invalidity.

Activity 9.5 Research and evidence-based practice

The Welshman and Walmsley article on the Learning Disability History research group website tells the story of community care for people with learning difficulties between 1948 and 2001. It explores how policy changed from controlling people in institutions to promoting their rights to be equal citizens. In a book called *Sans Everything*, Barbara Robb (1967) described her own experience of being poorly treated at a hospital. Robb launched a campaign to improve or close long-stay facilities. Not long afterwards, a nurse at a long-stay hospital for the mentally handicapped in Cardiff reported incidences of brutality and poor care. This was exposed to the *News of the World* and prompted an official inquiry. Its findings were highly critical of conditions, staff morale and management. In the 1980s there was increasing criticism and concern about the quality of long-term care for dependent people. There was also concern about the experiences of people leaving institutional care and being left to fend for themselves in the community.

Activity 9.6 Critical thinking and reflection

There are many potential answers to this activity. This is only a very brief reflection, but answers could range from external social structural issues (the financial provision for care of clients in homes and the resources required to support, train and supervise staff) to internal mental conceptions of self and clients, including the dehumanising effects of institutional care. The report suggests poor supervision and training of staff, partly a result of management failure. The individuals concerned may have never considered their own attitudes and values towards the people they work with; group practices and climate of fear may have prevented whistleblowing. The safeguards included internal management audits and inspection, professional codes of conduct, external inspection by the Care Quality Commission and the legal framework regarding abuse and assault. Fully engaging family and friends in care may also allow inspection of quality and provide staff with feedback. People with learning disabilities may still be considered by some people as less than adult and therefore with fewer rights to autonomy. Professionals are bound by their own codes and knowledge of the legal framework. As individuals, we need to be very critical of our own practice, examining our own assumptions and values to certain client groups so that we may identify practices that might seem normal, but are in fact abusive. The old concepts of clinical supervision and clinical governance have to have teeth.

Activity 9.7 Critical thinking and team working

As this activity has many potential discussion points, we will briefly address the *No Secrets* report (Department of Health, 2000). This report came about following serious incidents of abuse. Remember, this report predates the learning disabilities incidents at Cornwall Partnership Trust, Winterbourne View and Mid Staffs. The basis of the report is the Human Rights Act 1998, and it tries to ensure vulnerable adults are not abused through better interagency working. The primary aim is prevention of abuse in the first place, but if that fails, then there should be robust procedures in place to deal with it. Recent poor-quality care issues may indicate that the provisions of the *No Secrets* report have not been sufficiently robust.

Further reading

Broussine, E and Scarborough, K (2011) *Supporting People with Learning Disabilities in Health and Social Care.* London: SAGE.

Hardy, S et al. (2011) *Meeting the Health Needs of People with a Learning Disability.* London: RCN. Available online at: **http://www.rcn.org.uk/__data/assets/pdf_file/0004/78691/003024.pdf**

Trenoweth, S, Docherty, T, Franks, J, and Pearce, R (2011) *Nursing and Mental Health Care: An Introduction for all Fields of Practice.* Exeter: Learning Matters.

These three titles give essential background information.

Useful websites

www.bild.org.uk

The website for the British Institute for Learning Disabilities.

www.patient.co.uk

Search under 'For Professionals' for discussions on topics such as suicide, substance abuse and other mental health issues.

http://www.rcn.org.uk/development/practice/social_inclusion/learning_disabilities

http://www.rcn.org.uk/development/practice/social_inclusion/mental_health

Two Royal College of Nursing sites for learning disabilities and mental health – good resources and links.

Conclusion

Current issues and future directions

Throughout the book a recurrent theme seems to emerge. That theme is 'challenge'. There are so many challenges nurses face every day in delivering high-quality care in the face of issues, often seemingly beyond their individual control. The Nursing and Midwifery Council (NMC) exists to protect the public first and foremost through the application of professional standards. The protection afforded to individual nurses operates through their adherence to those standards. However, we have seen that this has not been enough to prevent some shocking lapses in the quality of care, as discussed, for example, in Chapters 1 and 9. The NMC highlights the personal and individual accountability of those on the register, but to stop there and blame individuals for those lapses in care demonstrates a lack of sociological imagination and an ignorance of complex psychological motivations and decision-making processes.

We would not wish to condone lapses by registered professionals. Individual accountability has to be a cornerstone of professional practice. In Chapter 2 it was noted that professional practice itself and the values we espouse need careful scrutiny. However, account has to be taken of the complex sociopolitical contexts and the psychosocial constructs that individual nurses experience in the creation of personal 'selves' as nurses. Chapters 3 and 5 discussed some of those constructs and ways of thinking. The giving of oneself as a nurse, engaging in what has been called 'emotional labour', requires a good deal of personal resources to deal with the stressors that care involves. Chapter 7 explored one of the main stressors, loss and death, in an attempt to encourage the building of personal resilience.

When poor-quality care is reported, a common knee-jerk reaction is to blame university-educated nurses, with calls to return to old-style ('golden-age') training. This is a mistake. The arguments are rehearsed in detail elsewhere (e.g. Shields et al., 2011). We should simply state that lapses in care call for more critical enquiry by nurses into practice, not less. This can only be done through a proper system of education in partnership between the NHS and the universities, in a situation where students are properly supported, supervised and encouraged by NHS staff who have the time, preparation and motivation to do this very important job. A few decades ago, Kath Melia (1984) pointed out the contradictory roles students (student vs worker) often have to play. It may well be the case that in too many clinical environments, which are facing budget restraints, this situation will not be eased soon.

In the many contributions to the debate about poor-quality care, there is often a distinct lack of sociological imagination. While individuals can be rightly criticised for giving poor care, the antecedents are to be found beyond the personal trouble of individual nurses and their patients, and can be classed as a public issue: that of the political, social and economic failures of the governing, managerial and administering classes over the past few decades.

Too Posh to Wash is the title of a recent publication on the condition of nursing (Beer, 2013) and reflects newspaper headlines and the Health Minister Jeremy Hunt's call to student nurses in March 2013. In it there is a range of contributions from various practitioners and experts on the delivery of care in the UK. They were asked to address various questions:

1. Why do we have lapses in nursing care and what needs to be done to prevent poor care in caring?
2. In striving for professionalism, have we over-qualified yet undertrained today's nurses? Are they too posh to wash? What mechanisms and support systems need to be in place to 'bring excellence' back into the profession?
3. Has the role of nurse leaders been devalued? Has respect for their knowledge and expertise and a desire to emulate them decreased?
4. Why have boards within both NHS and non-NHS organisations appeared to have failed to deliver the expected improvements in quality of care? Are board members unaware of the standards on their wards or in their care settings?

Various issues and solutions were raised but the answer to the title appears to be 'no', students are not too posh to wash. The myth of a golden age was shown to be just that – a myth. Menzies Lyth's (1960) paper was quoted and is still worth a read today.

Among the normative statements made, i.e. what nurses 'ought' and 'should' do, there was some attempt at analysis of underlying reasons for poor care. This included societal attitudes to ageing and caring, and technology and its effects on communication. There was no call however to return to apprenticeship training outside the university. This accords with the findings of the Willis Commission (2012).

What was striking was the almost passing references to systemic failures within the NHS around the structures for providing care. These failures are the responsibility of the governing political and managerial classes charged with running the NHS. While we are acknowledging ageing populations, increasing frailties and complex care needs, there is a requirement to examine the context of care; to examine what structures have been put in place to deliver care to increasing numbers of frail older people in acute hospitals and care homes. Student nurses in particular may be placed in clinical practices which are not conducive to compassionate care, and are often the least equipped to understand, analyse and bring about change.

Universities can support the development of critical thinking and underpinning knowledge but are almost powerless to affect this care context in which students find themselves. No amount of curricular changes emphasising compassion and caring will work if students continue to experience Melia's (1984) and Menzies Lyth's (1960) descriptions of the care environment.

Menzies Lyth (1960) argued that nurses experienced high levels of anxiety due to their work and that there was an absence in the hospital of any mechanism through which to *positively help the individual confront the anxiety provoking experiences.* The result was a set of defensiveness techniques, including the splitting up of the nurse–patient relationship. A more recent research report (Hillman et al., 2013) also reported *defensive practice*, resulting in an 'us and them' subject position regarding their patients as nurses felt the pressures of litigation, complaints and the pressing need to meet the managerial requirements of the organisation.

In the *Too Posh to Wash* document (Beer, 2013), three commentators pointed out the critical place that clinical practice experiences have which implicitly build upon the work of Menzies Lyth and Kath Melia. Professor David Sines argued (Beer, 2013) that there needs to be:

1. dynamic placement opportunities for students that expose and challenge them to confront the complexity of health and social care, within, between and across clinical care pathways, supported by a curriculum that is *wrapped around the patient's/user's real experience and journey*;
2. robust, enhanced and effective mentorship and preceptorship partnerships with our Trusts.

Sines goes on to argue:

> *Above all our next generation workforce requires access to expert mentorship and role models to nurture and inculcate excellence in practice and resilience in attitude to deliver optimal standards of care at all times, turning each patient encounter into a learning opportunity that leads to sustainable excellence.*
> (p. 15)

Again this is a key issue: *access to expert mentors.* Far too many students report the lack of both access and the quality of support in this area. Therefore this may, sadly, in the current context, be too idealistic. This may be borne out by Bradbury Jones et al. (2011), who reported that not all students have a positive experience, as also discussed by Lindop (1999), Levett-Jones and Lathlean (2008) and Levett-Jones et al. (2009). Maura Buchanan also focuses attention on the clinical environment:

> *I would argue that the main responsibility for failing standards lies not with nurse education, rather, with the clinical practice environment for which employers must take blame.*
> (Levett-Jones et al., 2009, p. 17)

Jenny Aston also points to deficiencies in the clinical environment:

> *With university based training [sic], considerable responsibility is left with the placement mentor to ensure that students have the necessary hands-on nursing skills. Many students have minimal one-to-one learning from their clinical mentors, who are busy with their own responsibilities, and have little or no protected time to teach the essential skills . . . University lecturers rarely have the time to visit, let alone work, in the clinical areas.*
> (Levett-Jones et al., 2009, p. 21)

Roy Lilley has often stated: *Fund the front line. Make it fun to work there, that way you will make Francis history* (**http://myemail.constantcontact.com/A-few-more-F-words.html?soid=1102665899193&a id=4IulmxtS6K4**). Nurses and nursing students have been criticised as lacking in compassion. No doubt this is true for some nurses. However, it is the lack of governance and poor clinical environments that both grow uncaring attitudes and fail to weed them out. Trust Boards, through excellent management, must implement strategies that ensure the front line is properly supported and developed.

Chapter 6 has outlined some of the key skills and challenges for nursing leaders. Sarah Parkin (2010) argues that much of leadership education does not clearly see the impending crises of unsustainable economic, business and political practice, has failed to see the wider picture and has failed to ask what leadership is for. We know we live in a messy world (Peccie, 1982; Morrall, 2009). If well-being is a goal, and if leadership involves vision and futures thinking, then working hard to reduce carbon emissions and engaging in sustainable lifestyles are visionary ambitions. Nursing leadership will be required to address climate change, which has become important for, and accepted by the UK government (see the Climate Change Act 2008 (Department for Environment Food and Rural Affairs, 2008), the Department of Health (2008a), and the National Health Service (National Health Service Sustainable Development Unit, 2009)). Indeed, Costello et al. (2009) argue that climate change has been identified as the biggest threat to global health of the twenty-first century. In this context, health workers have been urged by the British Medical Association (2008, 2011) to take action. International nursing organisations have also highlighted this as an imperative (American Nurses Association, 2008; Canadian Nurses Association, 2008, 2010; International Council of Nurses, 2008).

Some of the most pressing health issues facing us are international (World Health Organization, 2008). There are global threats to health and well-being from a wide range of economic, environmental and political issues, which we touched upon in Chapter 4. These health issues are particularly important for women and children (considered in Chapter 8), whose experiences of pregnancy, childbirth and child care are closely linked to the social and political situations they find themselves in. The United Nations Millennium Development Goals (2012) have rightly focused on maternal health, infant mortality and education for women as extremely important for global health gains.

We know also that economic inequality has direct health effects. The mortality rate for children under 5 is, in many countries, still far above the stated target of the Millennium Development Goals. We also know that political conflict has not gone away, leading us to understand that the world is ever more uncertain. Old beliefs in human progress and economic stability have been severely challenged and we are yet to construct a robust response. Globalisation results in large capital flows, labour movement and displacement, and the increasing dominance of transnational corporations on economic, social and political life. The demise of state power for the public good and its alignment with finance capital (Crouch, 2011) result in its increasing withdrawal from public services in many European countries. The transnational corporations and 'the markets' are two voices guiding politics. The current Eurozone crisis illustrates how politicians have to create polices that the international financial institutions feel are acceptable to them. Collier (2007) suggests that we have a bottom billion stuck in poverty, and the World Health Organization acknowledges wide health inequalities. Even for the rich, threats to survival are not domestic, but global. Perspectives are changing from local to global; the ethics of healthcare thus needs to be discussed in this context. The Millennium Development Goals also set a global policy framework.

Thus, there is an urgent need for healthcare professionals to address the sustainability of current politics, economics and social practices. The exact nature of that response is down to individuals. However, without some macro analysis we are in danger of leading ourselves into the dark. This then leads us to ask about our ethical responsibilities on a globalised world aiming at a *good life for all* (Ricoeur, 1992).

Many nurses have for a long time been pioneers for social action, acting on behalf of the poor, weak and vulnerable. That is their ethic. Peter Morrall (2009) has argued that we as health professionals and/or academics have an ethical responsibility to take individual, collegiate and organisational action with regard to the ills that affect human health and happiness.

However, taking a stand is hard. Ethics is hard and requires thinking. We may be the only sentient being on the planet who can think and reflect on our existence and the search for 'truth'. It may be that we have a special responsibility to think about our decisions and why we make them (Horowitz, 2011). But this may lead to 'moral distress' and moral responsibility by understanding the disparities in health. If we have responsibility, what does that mean? We may provoke moral distress, then what?

Nurse clinicians may experience moral distress when they are unable to translate their moral choices into moral action. The costs of unrelieved moral distress are high; ultimately, as with all unresolved professional conflicts, the quality of patient care suffers.

We hope this book has not only provided some material to reflect upon, but material that has been provocative as well. We have only been able to touch upon the many theories, concepts and philosophies that exist, so you will now need to make your own personal journey of discovery, debate and discussion in the building of your own personal nursing theory.

Bibliography

Abbott, P and Wallace, C (1990) *The Sociology of the Caring Professions*. London: Falmer Press.

Acheson Report (1998) *Independent Inquiry into Inequalities in Health*. London: The Stationery Office.

Adair, J (1973) *Action Centered Leadership*. New York: McGraw-Hill.

Advisory Council on the Misuse of Drugs (2008) *MDMA (Ecstasy): A Review of Its Harms and Classification Under the Misuse of Drugs Act 1971*. London: ACMD, Home Office.

Aked, J and Thompson, S (2011) *Five Ways to Wellbeing: New Applications, New Ways of Thinking*. NHS Confederation. New Economics Foundation (nef). Available online at: http://www.nhsconfed.org/Publications/reports/Pages/Five-ways-to-wellbeing.aspx

Allport, G (1954) *The Nature of Prejudice*. Cambridge, MA: Addison-Wesley.

American Nurses Association (ANA) (2008) *Global Climate Change*. Available online at: www.nursingworld.org

American Psychiatric Association (2000) *Diagnostic and Statistical Manual of Mental Disorders: DSM-IV-TR*, 4th edn. Washington, DC: American Psychiatric Association.

American Psychiatric Association (2013) *Diagnostic and Statistical Manual of Mental Disorders*, 5th edn. Arlington, VA: American Psychiatric Association.

Annandale, E and Field, D (2007) Socio-economic inequalities in health. In: Taylor, S and Field, D (eds) *Sociology of Health and Health Care*, 4th edn. Oxford: Blackwell.

Appleby, J (2013) *Spending on Health and Social Care over the Next 50 Years: Why Think Long Term?* London: The King's Fund.

Ariès, P (1981) *The Hour of Our Death*. Harmondsworth: Penguin.

Ashley, J (2013) NHS England is finally taking expert advice from the patients. *The Guardian* 7 October. Available online at: http://www.theguardian.com/commentisfree/2013/oct/06/nhs-england-patients-experts

Aylott, J, Brown, I, Copeland, R and Johnson, D (2008) *Tackling Obesities: The Foresight Report and Implications for Local Government*. Sheffield: Sheffield Hallam University. Available online at: www.idea.gov.uk/idk/aio/8268011

Bach, S and Ellis, P (2015) *Leadership, Management and Team Working in Nursing*, 2nd edn. London: SAGE Publications.

Bach, S and Grant, A (2015) *Communication and Interpersonal Skills for Nurses*, 3rd edn. London: SAGE Publications.

Baggot, R (2010) *Public Health Policy and Politics*. Basingstoke: Palgrave Macmillan.

Bandura, A (1977) Self-efficacy: toward a unifying theory of behavioral change. *Psychological Review*, 84: 191–215.

Bandura, A (1999) Moral disengagement in the perpetration of inhumanities. *Personality and Social Psychology Review*, 3: 193–209.

Bandura, A and Walters, R (1963) *Social Learning and Personality Development*. New York: Holt, Rinehart & Winston.

Banks, S (1998) *The Missing Link: Reflections on Philosophy and Spirit*. Edmonton: Lone Pine Publishing.

Barton, H and Grant, M (2006) A health map for the local human habitat. *Journal of the Royal Society for the Promotion of Health*, 126 (6): 252–261.

Basu, S and Stuckler, D (2013) *The Body Economic*. London: Allen Lane.

Baumann, Z (2000) *Liquid Modernity*. Cambridge: Polity.

BBC (2010) *Christopher Hitchens Talks to Jeremy Paxman. Newsnight* special, 29 November 2010. Available online at: http://news.bbc.co.uk/1/hi/9233571.stm

BBC (2011a) *Four Arrests After Patient Abuse Caught on Film.* 1 June 2011. Available online at: www.bbc.co.uk/news/uk-13548222

BBC (2011b) *Watchdog to Meet Over Care Concerns in Cornwall.* 21 June 2011. Available online at: http://tinyurl.com/lackofdignity

BBC (2011c) *UK Military Deaths in Afghanistan and Iraq.* July 2011. Available online at: www.bbc.co.uk/news/uk-10629358

BBC (2011d) *Cornwall Care Staff Suspended Over Abuse Allegations.* 2 December 2011. Available online at: www.bbc.co.uk/news/uk-england-cornwall-16003592

BBC (2014a) Clegg attacks NHS mental health care. 20 January 2014. Available online at: http://www.bbc.co.uk/news/health-25777429

BBC (2014b) *Nurses Warn of Mental Health Services Strain.* 23 November 2014. Available online at: http://www.bbc.co.uk/news/health-30150747

Beauchamp, T and Childress, J (2009) *Principles of Biomedical Ethics,* 6th edn. Oxford: Oxford University Press.

Becker, H (1997) *Outsiders.* New York: Free Press.

Beer, G. (ed.) (2013) *Too Posh to Wash? Reflections on the Future of Nursing.* Available online at: http://www.2020health.org/2020health/Publications/Publications-2013/Too-posh-to-wash.html

Belbin, M (2003) *Team Role Theory.* Available online at: www.belbin.com

Benner, P (1988) *The Primacy of Caring: Stress and Coping in Health and Illness.* Reading, MA: Addison-Wesley.

Bennis, W and Goldsmith, J (2003) Chapter 7. In: Bogle, J (ed.) (2009) *Enough! True Measures of Money, Business and Life.* Hoboken, NJ: Wiley, p. 159.

Benson, O and Stangroom, J (2006) *Why Truth Matters.* London: Continuum.

Bilton, T, Bonnett, K, Jones, P, Lawson, T, Skinner, D, Stanworth, M and Webster, A (2002) *Introductory Sociology,* 4th edn. Basingstoke: Palgrave Macmillan.

Bishop, V (2009) *Leadership for Nursing and Allied Health Professionals.* Maidenhead: McGraw Hill/Open University Press.

Bogle, J (2009) *Enough! True Measures of Money, Business and Life.* Hoboken, NJ: Wiley.

Boseley, S (2014) Two thirds of Britons with depression get no treatment. *The Guardian* 13 August. Available online at: http://www.theguardian.com/society/2014/aug/13/two-thirds-britons-not-treated-depression

Bowlby, J (1979) *The Making and Breaking of Affectional Bonds.* London: Tavistock Publications.

Bradbury Jones, C, Sambrook, S and Irvine, F (2011) Empowerment and being valued: a phenomenological study of nursing student's experiences of clinical practice. *Nurse Education Today,* 31: 368–372.

British Medical Association (BMA) Board of Science (2008) *Health Professionals Taking Action on Climate Change.* Available online at: www.bma.org.uk

British Medical Association (BMA) (2011) *The Health and Security Perspectives of Climate Change.* 17 October. Available online at: http://climatechange.bmj.com/statement

British Sociological Association (2010) *What Is Sociology?* Available online at: http://www.britsoc.co.uk/what-is-sociology.aspx

Canadian Nurses Association (CNA) (2008) *The Role of Nurses in Addressing Climate Change: A Background Paper.* Available online at: www.cna-aiic.ca

Canadian Nurses Association (CNA) (2010) *Climate Change and Health: A Position Statement.* Available online at: www.cna-aiic.ca

Capra, F (1982) *The Turning Point*. London: HarperCollins.

Care Quality Commission (CQC) (2014) *The State of Health Care and Adult Social Care in England 2013/14*. Available online at: www.cqc.org.uk

Carlisle, S (2001) Inequalities in health: contested explanations, shifting discourses and ambiguous polices. *Critical Public Health*, 11 (3): 267–281.

Carlson, NR, Buskist, W, Heth, CD and Schmaltz, R (2005) *Psychology: The Science of Behavior*, 3rd Canadian edn. Toronto: Pearson Education.

Carnevali, D (1984) *Diagnostic Reasoning in Nursing*. Philadelphia, PA: Lippincott.

Carper, B (1978) Fundamental patterns of knowing in nursing. *Advances in Nursing Science*, 1 (1): 13–24.

Carr-Saunders, A and Wilson, P (1933) *The Professions*. Oxford: Clarendon Press.

Centre for Maternal and Child Enquiries (CMACE) (2011) Saving mothers' lives. *British Journal of Obstetrics and Gynaecology*, 118 (suppl. 1): 1–203.

Chalmers, D J (1997) *The Conscious Mind: In Search of a Fundamental Theory*. Oxford: Oxford University Press.

Chambers, P (2010) Age and aging. In: Denny, E and Earle, S (eds) *Sociology for Nurses*, 2nd edn. Cambridge: Polity Press.

Chapman, J (2003) Public value: the missing ingredient in reform. In: Bentley, T and Wilsdon, J (eds) *The Adaptive State*. London: Demos.

Charlton, J (1998) *Nothing About Us Without Us*. Berkeley, CA: University of California Press.

Chartered Institute of Environmental Health (CIEH) (2011) *Are We Born to Lose?* Available online at: www.cieh.org/ehn/ehn3.aspx?id=37124

Chase, C (1995) The social context of critical care judgement. *Heart and Lung*, 24 (2): 154–162.

Clark, D (1997) *Growing a Team*. Available online at: www.nwlink.com/~donclark/leader/leadtem.html

Clinical Knowledge Summaries (CKS) (2011) *Depression, Ante and Post Natal*. Available online at: http://cks.nice.org.uk/depression-antenatal-and-postnatal

Cohen, P (2003) The Drug Prohibition Church and the adventure of reformation. *International Journal of Drug Policy*, 14 (2): 213–215. Available online at: http://tinyurl.com/9qfhl

Collier, P (2007) *The Bottom Billion: Why the Poorest Countries Are Failing and What Can Be Done About It*. Oxford: Oxford University Press.

Collins, M (2006) Taking a lead on stress: rank and relationship awareness in the NHS. *Journal of Nursing Management*, 14 (4): 310–317.

Cook, E (2010) Neglected hospital patients were left starving, sobbing and humiliated. *Daily Mirror*, 25 February. Available online at: www.mirror.co.uk/news/top-stories/2010/02/25/neglected-hospital-patients-were-left-starving- sobbing-humiliated-115875-22068295

Cooley, C (1902) *Human Nature and the Social Order*. New York: Scribner's.

Cornwell, J, Smith, P and Donaldson, J (2013) Forthcoming special issue – compassionate care – call for papers. *Nurse Education Today*, 33: 303–304.

Costello, A, Abbas, M, Allen, A, Ball, S, Bell, S, Bellamy, R, Friel, S, Groce, N, Johnson, A, Kett, M, Lee, M, Levy, C, Maslin, M, McCoy, D, McGuire, B, Montgomery, H, Napier, D, Pagel, C, Patel, J, de Oliveira, J A, Redclift, N, Rees, H, Rogger, D, Scott, J, Stephenson, J, Twigg, J, Wolff, J and Patterson, C (2009) Managing the health effects of climate change: *Lancet* and University College London Institute for Global Health Commission. *Lancet*, 373 (9676): 1693–1733.

Cottrill, K and Gary, L (2006) *How Soft Metrics Can Make Hard Choices Easier*. Harvard Business Publishing Newsletters. Available online at: http://hbr.org/product/how-soft-metrics-can-make-hard-choices-easier/an/P0601C-PDF-ENG

Cracknell, R (2010) The ageing population. Key issues for the new parliament 2010. *House of Commons Library Research*, page 44.

Crawford, R (1977) You are dangerous to your health: the ideology and politics of victim blaming. *International Journal of Health Services*, 4: 663–680.

Crouch, C (2011) *The Strange Non Death of Neoliberalism.* Cambridge: Polity.

Cumming, E and Henry, W (1961) *Growing Old: The Process of Disengagement.* New York: Basic Books.

Cunningham, G and Kitson, A (2000a) An evaluation of the RCN clinical leadership development programme: part 1. *Nursing Standard*, 15 (12): 34–37.

Cunningham, G and Kitson, A (2000b) An evaluation of the RCN clinical leadership development programme: part 2. *Nursing Standard*, 15 (13): 34–40.

Curtis, K (2013) 21st century challenges faced by nursing faculty in educating for compassionate practice: embodied interpretation of phenomenological data. *Nurse Education Today*, 33: 746–750.

Dahlgren, G and Whitehead, M (1991) *Policies and Strategies to Promote Social Equity in Health.* Stockholm: Institute for Futures Studies.

Davidson, A (2015) *Social Determinants of Health: A Comparative Approach.* Oxford: Oxford University Press.

Dawkins, R (2006) *The God Delusion.* London: Bantam Books.

Demers, A et al. (2002) in Davidson, A (2015) *Social Determinants of Health: A Comparative Approach.* Oxford: Oxford University Press, p. 239.

Dennis, CL and Hodnett, E (2007) *Psychosocial and Psychological Interventions for Treating Postpartum Depression.* Cochrane Review Issue 4. Chichester: John Wiley.

Dennis, T and Dennis, M (2006) *This Leadership Thing: The Usefulness Formula.* Occasional paper series. Healthcare Alliances. Available online at: www.healthcarealliances.co.uk

Dennis, T and Dennis, M (2011) *Good Organisations Are Good for You; Bad Organisations Can Harm You.* Occasional paper series. Healthcare Alliances. Available online at: www.healthcarealliances.co.uk

Department for Environment, Food and Rural Affairs (DEFRA) (2008) *Climate Change Act 2008.* London: HMSO.

Department of Health (1999) *Making a Difference: Strengthening the Contributions of Nursing, Midwifery and Health Visiting to Health and Healthcare.* Available online at: www.dh.gov.uk

Department of Health (2000) *No Secrets: Guidance on Protecting Vulnerable Adults in Care.* London: Department of Health.

Department of Health (DH) (2001a) *Seeking Consent: Working with People with LD.* London: Department of Health. Available online at: www.dh.gov.uk

Department of Health (2001b) *The Essence of Care.* London: Department of Health.

Department of Health (2001c) *Valuing People: A New Strategy for Learning Disability for the 21st Century.* London: Department of Health.

Department of Health (DH) (2008a) *Health Effects of Climate Change in the UK: An Update of the Department of Health Report, 2001/2002.* Available online at: www.dh.gov.uk/en/Publicationsandstatistics/Publications/PublicationsPolicyAndGuidance/DH_4007935

Department of Health (2008b) *The National End of Life Care Strategy.* London: Department of Health.

Department of Health (2009) *The NHS Constitution.* London: Department of Health

Department of Health (2010a) *Essence of Care 2010.* Available online at: https://www.gov.uk/government/publications/essence-of-care-2010

Department of Health (2010b) *Valuing People Now.* London: Department of Health.

Department of Health (DH) (2012a) *Liberating the NHS: No Decision About Me, Without Me. Government Response*. Available online at: https://www.gov.uk/government/uploads/system/uploads/attachment_data/file/216980/Liberating-the-NHS-No-decision-about-me-without-me-Government-response.pdf

Department of Health (2012b) *Compassion in Practice*. London: Department of Health.

Department of Health (2013) *Information: To Share or Not to Share? The Information Governance Review*. London: Department of Health.

Department of Health (DH) (2014) *Closing the Gap: Priorities for Essential Change in Mental Health*. Available online at: www.gov.uk

Department for Transport (DfT) (2011) *Reported Road Casualties in Great Britain: Annual Report 2010*. London: DfT.

Dilnot, A (2011) *Commission on Funding of Care and Support*. Available online at: www.dilnotcommission.dh.gov.uk

Directive 2005/36/EC of the European Parliament and of the Council of 7 September 2005 on the recognition of professional qualifications. *Official Journal of the European Union*, L255: 22–142.

Dorling, D (2014) *Inequality and the 1%*. London: Verso.

Doward, J (2014) England's child mental health services 'failing three quarters of kids'. *The Observer* 18 May. Available online at: http://www.theguardian.com/society/2014/may/18/child-mental-health-services-under-pressure

Drife, J (2005) Why mothers die. *Journal of the Royal College of Physicians Edinburgh*, 35: 322–336.

Drucker, P (1994) *Post-Capitalist Society*. Oxford: Butterworth-Heinemann.

Drugscope (2009) *Ecstasy*. Available online at: www.drugscope.org.uk/resources/drugsearch/drugsearch pages/ecstasy

Durkheim, E (1957) Professional ethics and civic morals. In: Morrall, P (ed.) (2001) *Sociology and Nursing*. London: Routledge.

Durkheim, E (1970; first published 1897) *Suicide: A Study in Sociology*. London: Routledge & Kegan Paul.

Dusheck, J (2002) The interpretation of genes. *Natural History*, 111 (8): 52–60.

Easton, M (2009) *Nutt Gets the Sack*. BBC News. 30 October. Available online at: www.bbc.co.uk/blogs/there porters/markeaston/2009/10/nutt_gets_the_sack.html

Edinburgh Napier University and NHS Lothian (2012) *Leadership in Compassionate Care Programme: Final Report*. Available online at: http://researchrepository.napier.ac.uk/5935/?utm_source=rss&utm_medium=rss&utm_campaign=leadership-in-compassionate-care-programme-final-report

Edgley, A, Timmons, S and Crosbie, B (2009) Desperately seeking sociology: nursing students' perceptions of sociology on nursing courses. *Nurse Education Today*, January 29 (1): 16–23.

Edmonstone, J (2009) Clinical leadership: the elephant in the room. *International Journal of Health Planning and Management*, 24: 290–305.

Elias, N (1969) *The Civilizing Process*, vol. I. *The History of Manners*. Oxford: Blackwell.

Elias, N (1982) *The Civilizing Process*, vol. II. *State Formation and Civilization*. Oxford: Blackwell.

Elstein, A, Shulman, L and Sprafka, S (1978) *Medical Problem Solving: An Analysis of Clinical Reasoning*. Cambridge, MA: Harvard University Press.

Enteman, W (1993) *Managerialism: The Emergence of a New Ideology*. Madison: University of Wisconsin Press.

Fahey, T, Montgomery, AA, Barnes, J and Protheroe, J (2003) Quality of care for elderly residents in nursing homes and elderly people living at home: controlled observational study. *BMJ*, March 15 326 (7389): 580.

Falk-Raphael, A (1994) The making of global citizenship. In: van Steenbergen, B (ed.) *The Condition of Citizenship.* London: SAGE.

Falk-Raphael, A (2006) Globalization and global health: toward nursing praxis in the global community. *Advances in Nursing Science,* 29 (1): 2–14.

Ferns, T and Chojnacka, I (2005) Angels and swingers, matrons and sinners: nursing stereotypes. *British Journal of Nursing,* 14 (19): 1028–1032.

Finfgeld-Connett, D (2008) Meta-synthesis of caring in nursing. *Journal of Clinical Nursing,* 17: 196–204.

Fiske, ST (2004) *Social Beings: A Core Motives Approach to Social Psychology.* New York: John Wiley.

Fiske, ST and Taylor, SE (1991) *Social Cognition,* 2nd edn. New York: McGraw-Hill.

Fitzsimons, P (1999) Managerialism and education. In: Peters, M, Ghiraldelli, P, Žarnić, B and Gibbons, A (eds) *The Encyclopaedia of Educational Philosophy and Theory.* Available online at: http://www.ffst.hr/ENCYCLOPAEDIA/doku.php?id=managerialism_and_education

Foucault, M (2007; first published in 1969) *The Archaeology of Knowledge.* London: Routledge.

Francis, R (2010) *Independent Inquiry into Care Provided by Mid Staffordshire NHS Foundation Trust January 2005–March 2009.* Available online at: www.midstaffsinquiry.com

Francis, R (2013) *The Mid Staffordshire NHS Foundation Trust Public Inquiry: Final Report.* London: Department of Health.

Freshwater, D (2002) *Therapeutic Nursing: Improving Patient Care Through Self Awareness and Reflection.* London: SAGE.

Freudenberger, H (1974) Staff burnout. *Journal of Social Issues,* 30: 159–166.

Friedson, E (1970) Chapter 5. In: Morrall, P (ed.) (2001) *Sociology and Nursing.* London: Routledge.

Fromm, E (2002; first published 1956) *The Sane Society.* Abingdon: Routledge Classics.

Gawande, A (2014) *Being Mortal: Illness, Medicine and What Matters in the End.* London: Profile.

Gerhardt, S (2010a) *The Selfish Society: How We All Forgot to Love One Another and Made Money Instead.* London: Simon & Schuster.

Gerhardt, S (2010b) *The Selfish Society.* RSA events. 22 April. www.thersa.org/events/audio-and-past-events/2010/the-selfish-society

Gill, D and Hatcher, S (2003) Antidepressants for depression in medical illness (Cochrane review). *The Cochrane Library,* Issue 1. Oxford: Update Software.

Gilligan, C (1982) *In a Different Voice.* Cambridge, MA: Harvard University Press.

Glaser, B and Strauss, A (1965) *Awareness of Dying.* Chicago: Aldine.

Glaser, B and Strauss, A (1968) *Time for Dying.* Chicago: Aldine.

Goffman, E (1959) *The Presentation of Self in Everyday Life.* London: Penguin.

Goffman, E (1963) *Stigma: Notes on the Management of Spoiled Identity.* Englewood Cliffs, NJ: Prentice Hall.

Goldacre, B (2008) *Bad Science.* London: Fourth Estate.

Goodman, B (2011a) The one dimensional state of (UK) nurse education. *Nurse Education Today,* 31 (8): 725–726.

Goodman, B (2011b) The sociological imagination, provocative pedagogy and scholarship: re-valuing thinking and writing in nurse education. *Nurse Education Today,* 31 (5): 427–428.

Goodman, B (2011c) The need for a 'sustainability curriculum' in nurse education. *Nurse Education Today,* 31 (8): 733–737.

Goodman, B (2011d) Leadership and management in critical care. Available online at: http://plymouth.academia.edu/bennygoodman/Talks/60148/leadership_and_mangement_in_critical_care

Goodman, B (2014) Risk, rationality and learning for compassionate care: the link between management practices and the lifeworld of nursing. *Nurse Education Today,* 34 (9): 1265–1268.

Goodman, B (2015) Climate change and ecological public health. *Nursing Standard,* 29 (24): 37–41.

Goodman, B and Clemow, R (2008) *Nursing and Working with Other People.* Exeter: Learning Matters.

Goodman, B and Clemow, R (2010) *Nursing and Collaborative Practice.* Exeter: Learning Matters.

Goodman, B and Richardson, J (2009) Climate change, sustainability and health in United Kingdom higher education: the challenges for nursing. In: Jones, P, Selby, D and Sterling, S (eds) *Sustainability Education: Perspectives and Practice Across Higher Education.* London: Earthscan.

Gordon, D, Mack, J, Lansley, S, Main, G, Nandy, S, Patsios, D and Pomati, M (2013) *The Impoverishment of the UK: PSE First Results: Living Standards.* Bristol: Bristol University.

Gregory, R (1972) Visual illusions. In Foss, B (ed.) *New Horizons in Psychology 1.* Harmondsworth: Penguin.

Griffiths, J, Speed, S, Horne, M and Keeley, P (2012) A caring professional attitude: what service users and carers seek in graduate nurses and the challenge for educators. *Nurse Education Today,* 32 (2): 121–127.

Groopman, J (2008) *How Doctors Think.* New York: Houghton Mifflin.

Gross, R and Kinnison, N (2013) *Psychology for Nurses and Allied Health Professionals,* 2nd edn. London: Hodder Arnold.

Guyatt, G, Oxman, A, Vist, G, Kunz, R, Flack-Ytter, Y, Alonso-Coello, P and Schunemann, H (2008) GRADE: an emerging consensus on rating quality of evidence and strength of recommendations. *British Medical Journal,* 336 (7650): 924–926.

Gyngell, K (2009) *The Phoney War on Drugs.* London: Centre for Policy Studies.

Habermas, J (1984) *The Theory of Communicative Action,* vols 1 and 2. Boston, MA: Beacon Press.

Hagell, E (1989) Nursing knowledge: women's knowledge. A sociological perspective. *Journal of Advanced Nursing,* 14: 226–233.

Hamilton, C (2003) *Growth Fetish.* London: Pluto Press.

Hamilton, C (2010) *Requiem for a Species.* London: Earthscan.

Hamm, R M (1988) Clinical intuition and clinical analysis: expertise and the cognitive continuum. In: Dowie, J and Elstein, A (eds) *Professional Judgment: A Reader in Clinical Decision Making.* Cambridge: Cambridge University Press, pp. 78–105.

Haney, C, Banks, WC and Zimbardo, PG (1973) Study of prisoners and guards in a simulated prison. *Naval Research Reviews,* 9: 1–17.

Hannon, L and Clift, J (2011) *General Hospital Care for People with Learning Disabilities.* Chichester: Wiley Blackwell.

Haralambos, M and Holborn, M (2013) *Haralambos and Holborn: Sociology Themes and Perspectives.* London: Harper Collins.

Health and Safety Executive (2011) *Work Related Injuries and Ill Health in Construction.* Available online at: www.hse.gov.uk/statistics/industry/construction/index.htm

Healthcare Commission (2007) *Investigation into the Service for People with Learning Disabilities Provided by Sutton and Merton Primary Care Trust.* January. London: Healthcare Commission.

Healthcare Commission and CSCI (Commission for Social Care Inspection) (2006) *Joint Investigation into the Provision of Services for People with Learning Disabilities at Cornwall Partnership NHS Trust.* July. London: Healthcare Commission and CSCI.

Helman, C (2007) *Culture, Health and Illness,* 5th edn. London: Hodder Arnold.

Henderson, V (1966) *The Nature of Nursing.* New York: Macmillan.

Hewison, A and Griffiths, M (2004) Leadership development in healthcare: a word of caution. *Journal of Health Organisation and Management,* 18 (6): 464–473.

Hill, M (2011) Care Quality Commission hit by 'no confidence' petition. *BBC News,* 29 June. Available online at: http://tinyurl.com/CQCnoconfidence

Hill, T (2010) How clinicians make (or avoid) moral judgments of patients: implications of the evidence for relationships and research. *Philosophy, Ethics and Humanities in Medicine,* 5 (11).

Hillman, A, Tadd, W, Calnan, S, Calnan, M, Bayer, A and Read, S (2013) Risk, governance and the experience of care. *Sociology of Health and Illness,* 35 (6): 939–955.

Hitchens, C (2007) *God Is Not Great: How Religion Poisons Everything.* New York: Twelve Books.

Hochschild, A (1983) *The Managed Heart.* Berkeley, CA: University of California Press.

Hofling, CK, Brotzman, E, Dalrymple, S, Graves, N and Pierce, CM (1966) An experimental study of nurse–physician relationships. *Journal of Nervous and Mental Disease,* 143: 171–180.

Holland, J (2003) Cited in Darman, J, Out of the club, onto the couch. *Newsweek,* 5 December. Available online at: www.mdma. net/psychotherapy/index.html

Home Office (2014) *Drugs: International Comparisons.* Available online at: https://www.gov.uk/government/publications

Hood, C (1991) A public management for all seasons. *Public Administration,* 69 (1): 3–19.

Hoopes, J (2003) *False Prophets: The Gurus Who Created Modern Management and Why Their Ideas Are Bad for Business.* New York: Basic Books.

Hopkins, R (2008) *The Transition Handbook.* Totnes: Green Books.

Horowitz, D (2011) *We Need a 'Moral Operating System'.* Available online at: www.ted.com/talks/damon_horowitz.html

Horton, R, Beaglehole, R, Bonita, R, Raeburn, J, McKee, M and Wall, S (2014) From public health to planetary health: a manifesto. *The Lancet,* 383: 847.

House, A (2003) Defining, recognising and managing depression. *Practical Neurology,* 3: 196–203.

House of Commons, Science and Technology Committee (2006) *Drug Classification: Making a Hash of It?* Available online at: www.publications.parliament.uk/pa/cm200506/cmselect/cmsctech/1031/1031.pdf

Hunt, S and Symonds, A (1995) *The Social Meaning of Midwifery.* Basingstoke: Macmillan.

Husserl, E. (1970; original 1936) *The Crisis of European Sciences and Transcendental Phenomenology.* Evanston: NorthWestern University Press.

Hutchinson, M and Jackson, D (2013) Transformational leadership in nursing: towards a more critical interpretation. *Nursing Inquiry,* 20 (1) 11–22.

Hyland, M and Donaldson, M (1989) *Psychological Care in Nursing Practice.* London: Scutari Press.

Illich, I (1975) *Medical Nemesis.* London: Calder and Boyars.

Illich, I (1976) *Limits to Medicine: Medical Nemesis, the Expropriation of Health.* London: Marion Boyars.

International Council of Nurses (ICN) (2008) *Nurses, Climate Change and Health: A Position Statement.* Available online at: www.icn.ch/images/stories/documents/publications/position_statements/E08_Nurses_Climate_Change_Health.pdf

Jackson, T (2009) *Prosperity without Growth.* London: Earthscan.

James, N (1993) Divisions of emotional labour: disclosure and cancer. In: Fineman, S (ed.) *Emotion in Organisations.* London: SAGE.

Jeffery, R (1979) Normal rubbish: deviant patients in casualty departments. *Sociology of Health and Illness,* 1 (1): 90–107.

Johnson, M and Webb, C (1995) Rediscovering the unpopular patient. *Journal of Advanced Nursing*, 21 (3): 466–475.

Jones, S (2009) Cited in: Alleyne, R and Devlin, K. Genetic research in a 'blind alley' in search for cures for common diseases. *The Telegraph*. Available online at: www.telegraph.co.uk/health/healthnews/5189873/Genetic-research-in-a-blind-alley-in-search-for-cures-for-common-diseases.html

Jourard, S M (1966) An exploratory study of body-accessibility. *British Journal of Social and Clinical Psychology*, 5: 221–231.

Kahneman, D (2011) *Thinking Fast and Slow*. Basingstoke: MacMillan.

Kahneman, D and Tversky, A (1996) On the reality of cognitive illusions. *Psychological Review*, 103 (3): 582–591.

Kastenbaum, R (2001) *Death, Society and Human Experience*, 7th edn. Boston, MA: Allyn & Bacon.

Katz, A and Alegria, M (2003) The clinical encounter as local moral world: shifts of assumptions and transformation in relational context. *Social Science and Medicine*, 68 (7): 1238–1246.

Katzenbach, J and Smith, D (1993) The discipline of teams. *Harvard Business Review*, 71: 111–146.

Kellehear, A (1990) *Dying of Cancer: The Final Year of Life*. London: Harwood.

Kelly, GA (1955) *The Psychology of Personal Constructs* (vols 1 and 2). New York: Norton.

Kent, A (2008) Improving care of people with learning disabilities. *Nursing Times*, 104 (5): 32–33.

King's Fund (2011) *The Future of Leadership and Management in the NHS: No More Heroes*. London: The King's Fund.

Kmietowicz, Z (2009) Home secretary accused of bullying drugs adviser over comments about ecstasy. *British Medical Journal*, 338: b612.

Kobasa, SC (1979) Stressful life events, personality, and health: an inquiry into hardiness. *Journal of Personality and Social Psychology*, 37: 1–11.

Kouzes, J and Posner, B (2011) *The Five Practices of Exemplary Leadership*, 2nd edn. San Francisco, CA: Wiley.

Kübler-Ross, E (1969) *On Death and Dying*. New York: Macmillan.

Lagos, TG (2002) *Global Citizenship: Towards a Definition*. Available online at: http://depts.washington.edu/gcp/pdf/globalcitizenship.pdf

Lang, T and Rayner, G (2012) Ecological public health: the 21st century's big idea? *British Medical Journal* 345: e5466.

Lawler, J (1991) *Behind the Screens: Nursing, Somology, and the Problem of the Body*. Melbourne: Churchill Livingstone.

Lawton, J (2000) *The Dying Process: Patients' Experiences of Palliative Care*. London: Routledge.

Lawton, J (2002) Contemporary hospice care: the sequestration of the unbounded body and 'dirty dying' in England. In: Nettleton, S and Gustaffson, U (eds) *The Sociology of Health and Illness*. Cambridge: Polity Press.

Lazarus, RS and Folkman, S (1984) *Stress, Appraisal and Coping*. New York: Springer.

Leader, D (2011) *What Is Madness?* Talk at the Royal Society of Arts. 21 October. Available online at: www.thersa.org/events

Lees, A, Meyer, E and Rafferty, J (2013) From Menzies Lyth to Munro: the problem of managerialism. *British Journal of Social Work*, 43: 542–558.

Leininger, M (1995) *Transcultural Nursing: Concepts, Theories, Research and Practice*. Columbus, OH: McGraw-Hill College Custom Series.

Lessa, I (2006) Discursive struggles within social welfare: restaging teen motherhood. *British Journal of Social Work*, 36 (2): 283–298.

Levett-Jones, T and Lathlean, J (2008) Belongingness: a prerequisite for nursing students' clinical learning. *Nurse Education in Practice*, 8: 103–111.

Levett-Jones, T, Lathlean, J, Higgins, I and McMillan, M (2009) Staff–student relationships and their impact on nursing students' belongingness and learning. *Journal of Advanced Nursing*, 65 (2): 316–324.

Lewin, K (1948) *Resolving Social Conflicts*. New York: Harper & Row.

Lindop, E (1999) A comparative study of stress between pre- and post-Project 2000 students. *Journal of Advanced Nursing*, 29 (4): 967–973.

Liu, Y-E, Norman, IJ and While, A (2012) Nurses' attitudes towards older people: a systematic review. *International Journal of Nursing Studies*, 50 (9): 1271–1282.

LoBindo-Wood, G and Haber, J (1998) *Nursing Research: Methods, Critical Appraisal and Utilisation*, 4th edn. St Louis, MO: Mosby.

London Weekend Television (1983) *Breadline Britain* (a booklet accompanying the television series). London: LWT.

Lorber, J (1975) Good patients and problem patients: conformity and deviance in a general hospital. *Journal of Health and Social Behaviour*, 16 (2): 213–225.

Lustman, P and Anderson, R (2002) Depression in adults with diabetes. *Psychiatric Times*, January 19 (1).

Lyons, J (1977) *Semantics*, vol. 2. Cambridge: Cambridge University Press.

MacCoun, R and Reuter, P (2008) The implicit rules of evidence-based drug policy: a US perspective. *International Journal of Drug Policy*, 19: 231–232.

Mackenbach, P (2012) The persistence of health inequalities in modern welfare states. *Social Science and Medicine*, 75 (4): 761–769.

MacIntosh, J (1977) *Communication and Awareness in a Cancer Ward*. London: Croom Helm.

MacKay, M (2010) Why nursing has not embraced the clinician-scientist role. *Nursing Philosophy*, 10: 287–296.

Marmot, M (2010) *Fair Society, Healthy Lives. The Marmot Review. Strategic Review of Health Inequalities in England Post 2010*. Available online at: www.marmotreview.org

Maslach, C and Jackson, S (1986) *The Maslach Burn-Out Inventory Manual*, 2nd edn. Palo Alto, CA: Consulting Psychologists Press.

Maslow, A (1954) *Motivation and Personality*. New York: Harper.

Mason, P (2012) Global unrest: how the revolution went viral (extract from *Why It's Kicking Off Everywhere: The New Global Revolutions*. London: Verso). *The Guardian* 3 January. Available online at: www.guardian.co.uk/world/2012/jan/03/how-the-revolution-went-viral

McCormack, B and Corner, J (2003) Learning together: caring together. *Health Education Journal*, 62 (3): 195–197.

McKinnon, J (2014) Pursuing concordance: moving away from paternalism. *British Journal of Nursing*, 23 (12): 677–684.

McLuhan, M (1964) *Understanding Media: The Extensions of Man*. Cambridge, MA: MIT Press.

McVicar, A (2003) Workplace stress in nursing: a literature review. *Journal of Advanced Nursing*, 44 (6): 633–642.

Melia, K (1984) Student nurses' construction of occupational socialisation. *Sociology of Health and Illness*, 6 (2): 132–151.

Melia, K (1987) *Learning and Working: The Occupational Socialization of Nurses*. London: Tavistock.

Mencap (2007) *Death by Indifference*. Available online at: www.mencap.org.uk/node/5863

Mencap (2011) *Investigation Reveals 74 Deaths in Care*. 3 January. Available online at: www.mencap.org.uk/guardian_investigation

Menzies Lyth, I (1960) The functioning of social systems as a defence against anxiety. *Human Relations*, 13 (2): 95–121.

Michael, J (2008) *Healthcare for All: Report of the Independent Inquiry into Access to Healthcare for People with Learning Disabilities.* London: Department of Health.

Milgram, S (1963) Behavioral study of obedience. *Journal of Abnormal and Social Psychology*, 67 (4): 371–378.

Milgram, S (1974) *Obedience and Authority.* New York: Harper Torch Books.

Ministry of Health (1957) *Report on Confidential Enquiries into Maternal Deaths in England and Wales, 1952–54. Reports on Public Health and Medical Subjects No. 97.* London: HMSO.

Moerman, D (2003) *Meaning, Medicine and the Placebo Effect.* Cambridge Studies in Medical Anthropology (no. 9). Dearborn, MI: University of Michigan – Dearborn.

Monbiot, G (2011) Daniel Kahneman: how cognitive illusions blind us to reason. *The Observer*, 30 October. Available online at: www.guardian.co.uk/science/2011/oct/30/daniel-kahneman-cognitive-illusion-extract

Monbiot, G (2014) The age of loneliness is killing us. *The Guardian* 15 October. Available online at: http://www.theguardian.com/commentisfree/2014/oct/14/age-of-loneliness-killing-us

Montgomery, B and Dossey, L (2008) *Holistic Nursing: A Handbook for Practice.* London: Jones and Bartlett.

Mooney, C (2000) *Theories of Childhood: An Introduction to Dewey, Montessori, Erikson, Piaget and Vygotsky.* St Paul, MN: Redleaf Press.

Moos, RH and Schaefer, JA (1984) The crisis of physical illness: an overview and conceptual approach. In: Moos, RH (ed.) *Coping with Physical Illness: New Perspectives*, vol. 2. New York: Plenum Press, pp. 3–25.

Morrall, P (2001) *Sociology and Nursing.* London: Routledge.

Morrall, P (2009) *Sociology and Health.* London: Routledge.

Morrison, P and Burnard, P (1997) *Caring and Communicating: The Interpersonal Relationship in Nursing.* London: Macmillan.

Mulgan, G (2006) *Good and Bad Power.* London: Allen Lane.

Mulholland, J (1997) The sociology in nursing debate. *Journal of Advanced Nursing*, 25: 844–852.

Murray, K (2012) How doctors choose to die. *The Guardian* 8 February. Available online at: www.guardian.co.uk/society/2012/feb/08/how-doctors-choose-die

National Centre for Social Research (2010) *British Social Attitudes Survey.* Available online at: http://discover.ukdataservice.ac.uk/catalogue/?sn=6969&type=Data%20catalogue

National Collaborating Centre for Mental Health (2004) *Depression: Management of Depression in Primary and Secondary Care.* London: National Institute for Health and Clinical Excellence.

National Collaborating Centre for Mental Health (2007) *Antenatal and Postnatal Mental Health: The NICE Guideline on Clinical Management and Service Guidance* (full NICE guideline). London: National Institute for Health and Clinical Excellence.

National Health Service Sustainable Development Unit (NHS SDU) (2009) *Saving Carbon, Improving Health: NHS Carbon Reduction Strategy for England.* Available online at: www.sdu.nhs.uk/documents/publications/1237308334_qylG_saving_carbon,_improving_health_nhs_carbon_reducti.pdf

National Institute on Drug Abuse (2006) *MDMA (Ecstasy) Abuse.* Research Report series. March. Available online at: www.drugabuse.gov/publications/research-reports/mdma-ecstasy-abuse

National Institute for Health and Care Excellence (NICE) (2014) *NICE Confirms Midwife-Led Care During Labour Is Safest for Women with Straightforward Pregnancies.* Available online at: http://www.nice.org.uk/news/press-and-media/midwife-care-during-labour-safest-women-straightforward-pregnancies

Newell, R (2000) *Body Image and Disfigurement Care*. London: Routledge.

NSPCC (2014) *People Who Abuse Children: An NSPCC Research Briefing*. London: NSPCC.

Nursing and Midwifery Council (2008) *The Code: Standards of Conduct, Performance and Ethics for Nurses and Midwives*. Available online at: www.nmc-uk.org/Documents/Standards/The-code-A4-20100406.pdf

Nursing and Midwifery Council (2010) *Standards for Pre-registration Nursing Education*. Available online at: http://standards.nmc-uk.org

Nutt, D, King, L, Saulsbury, W and Blakemore, C (2007a) Development of a rational scale to assess the harm of drugs of potential misuse. *The Lancet*, 369 (9566): 1047.

Nutt, D, King, L, Saulsbury, W and Blakemore, C (2007b) Scientists want new drug rankings. *BBC News*. 23 March. Available online at: http://news.bbc.co.uk/1/hi/health/6474053.stm?ls#drugs

Oakley, A (1979) *Becoming a Mother*. Oxford: Martin Robertson. (Also published under the title *From Here to Maternity* (1981) Harmondsworth: Penguin.)

Oakley, A (1980) *Women Confined: Towards a Sociology of Childbirth*. Oxford: Martin Robertson.

Oakley, A (1984) *The Captured Womb: A History of the Medical Care of Pregnant Women*. Oxford: Basil Blackwell.

Office for National Statistics (ONS) (2005) *Mortality Statistics*. London: ONS.

Office for National Statistics (2009) *Life Expectancy at Birth Remains Highest in the South of England*. Available online at: http://aqmen.ac.uk/sites/default/files/ONS_News_Release.pdf

Oreskes, N and Conway, E (2010) *Merchants of Doubt*. New York: Bloomsbury.

Ottersen, O, Dasgupta, J, Blouin, C, Buss, P, Chongsuvivatwong, V, Frenk, J, Fukuda-Parr, S, Gawanas, B, Giacaman, R, Gyapong, J, Leaning, J, Marmot, M, McNeill, D, Mongella, G, Moyo, N, Mogedal, S, Ntsaluba, A, Ooms, G, Bjertness, E, Lie, A, Moon, S, Roalkvam, S, Sandberg, K and Scheel, I (2014) The Lancet-University of Oslo Commission on Global Governance for Health. The political origins of health inequity: prospects for change. *The Lancet*, 383: 630–667.

Palmieri, P, Peterson, L and Ford, E (2007) Technological iatrogenesis: new risks force heightened management awareness. *Journal of Healthcare Risk Management*, 27 (4): 19–24.

Parkes, C M (1972) *Bereavement: Studies of Grief in Adult Life*. Harmondsworth: Penguin.

Parkin, S (2010) *The Positive Deviant: Sustainability Leadership in a Perverse World*. London: Earthscan.

Parliamentary and Health Ombudsman (2009) *Six Lives: The Provision of Public Services to People with Learning Disabilities*. Norwich: The Stationery Office.

Parse, RR (1981) *Man–Living–Health: A Theory of Nursing*. New York: John Wiley.

Parsons, T (1951) *The Social System*. Glencoe, IL: Free Press.

Parsons, T (1955) The American family: its relations to personality and the social structure. In: Parsons, T and Bales, RF (eds) *Family, Socialization and Interaction Process*. New York: Free Press.

Peccie, A (1982) *One Hundred Pages for the Future: Reflections of the President of the Club of Rome*. London: Futura.

Perfetti, J, Clark, R and Fillmore, C M (2004) Postpartum depression: identification, screening, and treatment. *Wisconsin Medical Journal*, 103 (6): 56–63.

Perrone, D (2005) Drug set and setting: the neglected factors of the US response to club drugs. Paper presented at the annual meeting of the American Society of Criminology, Royal York, Toronto, 15 November.

Perry, P (2014) Loneliness is killing us: we must start treating this disease. *The Guardian* 17 February. Available online at: http://www.theguardian.com/commentisfree/2014/feb/17/loneliness-report-bigger-killer-obesity-lonely-people

Pescosolido, B (2000) Rethinking models of health and illness behaviour. In: Kelner, M, Wellman, B, Pescosolido, B and Saks, M (eds) *Complementary and Alternative Medicine: Challenge and Change.* Amsterdam: Harwood Academic Publishers.

Pielke, R (2010) *The Climate Fix: What Scientists and Politicians Won't Tell You About Global Warming.* New York: Basic Books.

Poverty and Social Exclusion (2013) *Going Backwards 1983–2012.* Available online at: http://www.poverty. ac.uk/pse-research/going-backwards-1983-2012

Preston, D (2001) The rise of managerialism. In: Peters, M, Ghiraldelli, P, Žarnić, B and Gibbons, A (eds) *The Encyclopaedia of Educational Philosophy and Theory.* Available online at: http://eepat.net/doku. php?id=the_rise_of_managerialism&s[]=rise&s[]=managerialism

Prout, A and Hallett, C (eds) (2003) *Hearing the Voices of Children: Social Policy for a New Century.* London: Falmer Press.

Public Health England (2013) *What We Now Know 2013.* London: Public Health England.

Riahi, S (2011) Role stress amongst nurses at the workplace: concept analysis. *Journal of Nursing Management,* 6: 721–731.

Ricaurte, G, Yuan, J, Hatzidimitriou, G, Cord, B and McCann, U (2002) Severe dopaminergic neurotoxicity in primates after a common recreational dose regimen of MDMA (ecstasy). *Science,* September (retracted 2003). Available online at: www.mdma.net/toxicity/ricaurte.html

Ricoeur, P (1992) *Oneself as Another.* Chicago, IL: The University of Chicago Press.

Ridley, M (2003) *Nature via Nurture: Genes, Experience, and What Makes Us Human.* London: HarperCollins.

Rittel, H W J and Webber, M (1973) Dilemmas in a general theory of planning. *Policy Science,* 4: 155–159.

Robb, B (1967) *Sans Everything.* London: Nelson.

Robb, M (2004) The end of paternalism? *Nursing Management,* 10 (10): 32–35.

Roberts, I and Edwards, P (2010) *The Energy Glut.* London: Zed Books.

Rogers, C (1961) *On Becoming a Person.* Boston, MA: Houghton Mifflin.

Rogers, ME (1970) *An Introduction to the Theoretical Basis of Nursing.* Philadelphia, PA: F.A. Davis.

Rolfe, G (2010) A reply to 'Why nursing has not embraced the clinician-scientist role' by Martha MacKay: nursing science and the post-modern menace. *Nursing Philosophy,* 11: 136–140.

Rolfe, G (2011) C. Wright Mills on intellectual craftsmanship. *Nurse Education Today,* 31 (2): 115–116.

Roper, N, Logan, W and Tierney, A (2000) *The Roper Logan and Tierney Model of Nursing.* Edinburgh: Churchill Livingstone.

Roy, C (1980) The Roy adaptation model. In: Riehl, JP and Roy, C (eds) *Conceptual Models for Nursing Practice.* Norwalk, CT: Appleton-Century Crofts.

Royal College of Midwives (RCM) (2011a) Campaign for normal birth. Available online at: www. rcmnormalbirth.org.uk

Royal College of Midwives (2011b) RCM report shows looming crisis for UK maternity services. Available online at: www.rcm.org.uk/college/about/media-centre/press-releases/rcm-report-shows-looming-crisis-for-uk-maternity-services-23-11-11/?locale=en

Royal College of Midwives (2011c) *State of Maternity Services Report.* Available online at: www.rcm.org.uk/ college/policy-practice/government-policy/state-of-maternity-services/?locale=en

Royal College of Nursing (RCN) (2003) *Defining Nursing.* London: RCN.

Royal College of Nursing (2010) *Care Homes under Pressure. RCN Policy Report 04/2010. An England Report.* London: RCN.

Royal College of Nursing (2011a) *Meeting the Health Needs of People with Learning Disabilities*. London: RCN.

Royal College of Nursing (2011b) *Fears Over Quality Care Revealed by Nurses*. February 2011. Available online at: www.rcn.org.uk/newsevents/press_releases/uk/fears_over_quality_care_revealed_by_nurses

Royal College of Nursing (2014) *Safeguarding Children and Young People: Every Nurse's Responsibility*. Available online at: http://www.rcn.org.uk/__data/assets/pdf_file/0004/78583/004542.pdf

Royal College of Psychiatrists (2010) *No Health Without Mental Health: The Case for Action*. Available online at: www.rcpsych.ac.uk/quality/quality,accreditationaudit/nohealthwithout.aspx

Running, A and Turnbeaugh, E (2011) Oncology pain and complementary therapy. *Clinical Journal of Oncology Nursing*, 15 (4): 374–379.

Sackett, D, Rosenberg, W, Muir Gray, J, Haynes, B and Richardson, WS (1996) Evidence based medicine: what it is and what it is not. *British Medical Journal*, 312 (7023).

Sandel, M (2012) *What Money Can't Buy: The Moral Limits of Markets*. London: Allen Lane.

Sargent, C (2006) *From Buddy to Boss: Effective Fire Service Leadership*. Tulsa, OK: PennWell.

Scambler, G (2012) *GBH: Greedy Bastards Hypothesis and Health Inequalities*. Available online at: https://grahamscambler.wordpress.com/2012/11/04/gbh-greedy-bastards-and-health-inequalities

Schmitt, T, Sims-Giddens, S and Booth, R (2012) Social media use in nursing education. OJIN: The Online Journal of Issues in Nursing (17) 3: Manuscript 2.

Seligman, MEP (1975) *Helplessness: On Depression, Development, and Death*. San Francisco: WH Freeman.

Selye, H (1956) *The Stress of Life*. New York: McGraw-Hill.

Shaputis, K (2004) *The Crowded Nest Syndrome: Surviving the Return of Adult Children*. Olympia, WA: Clutter Fairy Publishing.

Sharp, K (1994) Sociology and the nursing curriculum: a note of caution. *Journal of Advanced Nursing*, 20: 391–395.

Sharp, K (1995) Sociology in nurse education: help or hindrance? *Nursing Times*, 91 (20): 34–35.

Sharp, K (2010) Chapter 1, What is sociology? In: Denny, E and Earle, S (eds) *Sociology for Nurses*, 2nd edn. Cambridge: Polity.

Sheaff, M (2005) *Sociology and Healthcare: An Introduction for Nurses, Midwives and Allied Health Professionals*. Maidenhead: Open University Press.

Shields, L, Morrall, P, Goodman B, Purcell, C and Watson, R (2011) Care to be a nurse? Reflections on a radio broadcast and its ramifications for nursing today. *Nurse Education Today*, 32 (5): 614–617.

SIGN (2002) *Postnatal Depression and Puerperal Psychosis*. Edinburgh: Scottish Intercollegiate Guidelines Network. Available online at: www.sign.ac.uk

Singh, S and Ernst, E (2008) *Trick or Treatment: Alternative Medicine on Trial*. London: Bantam Press.

Siviter, B (2002) Personal interview of Nancy Roper at RCN Congress, Association of Nursing Students, reported in fall edition *The Answer* (RCN).

Smith, P (1992) *The Emotional Labour of Nursing*. London: Macmillan.

Smith, P (2012) *The Emotional Labour of Nursing Revisited: Can Nurses Still Care?* Basingstoke: Palgrave Macmillan.

Smith, P and Gray, B (2001) Reassessing the notion of emotional labour in student nurse education: role of lecturers and mentors in a time of change. *Nurse Education Today*, 21: 230–237.

Snowdon, C (2010) *The Spirit Level Delusion*. London: Little Dice Books.

Solvoli, B and Heggen, K (2010) Teaching and learning care: exploring nursing students' clinical practice. *Nurse Education Today*, 30 (1): 73–77.

Sparrow, B, Liu, J and Wegner, D (2011) Google effects on memory: cognitive consequences of having information at our fingertips. *Science*, 333 (6043): 776–778.

Standing, M (2008) Clinical judgement and decision-making in nursing: nine modes of practice in a revised cognitive continuum. *Journal of Advanced Nursing*, 62: 124–134.

Standing, M (2013) *Clinical Judgement and Decision Making for Nursing Students*, 2nd edn. London: SAGE Publications.

Stewart, R, Hargreaves, K and Oliver, S (2005) Evidence informed policy making for health communication. *Health Education Journal*, 64 (2): 120–128.

Stockwell, F (1972) *The Unpopular Patient*. London: RCN Publications.

Stroebe, M and Schut, H (1999) The dual process model of coping with bereavement: rationale and description. *Death Studies*, 23: 197–224.

Sudnow, D (1967) *Passing On: The Social Organisation of Dying*. New York: Prentice Hall.

Sullivan, E (2002) Nursing and feminism: an uneasy alliance. *Journal of Professional Nursing*, 18 (4): 183–184.

Thaler, R and Sunstein, C (2008) *Nudge: Improving Decisions about Health, Wealth and Happiness*. New Haven, CT: Yale University Press.

The Guardian (2014) I love working in mental health – but I can't do a good job on a shoestring. 1 December 2014. Available online at: http://www.theguardian.com/healthcare-network/views-from-the-nhs-front-line/2014/dec/01/mental-health-psychologist-resources-nhs

The Stationery Office (TSO) (2013) *The Care Bill Explained. Including a Response to Consultation and Pre-legislative Scrutiny on the Draft Care and Support Bill*. Available online at: https://www.gov.uk/government/uploads/system/uploads/attachment_data/file/228864/8627.pdf

Theodosius, C (2008) *Emotional Labour in Health Care: The Unmanaged Heart of Nursing*. Abingdon: Taylor and Francis.

Thurtle, V (1995) Post-natal depression: the relevance of sociological approaches. *Journal of Advanced Nursing*, 22 (3): 416–424.

Tillett, R (2003) The patient within – psychopathology in the helping professions. *Advances in Psychiatric Treatment*, 9: 272–279.

Timmermans, S (1998) Social death as a self-fulfilling prophecy: David Sudnow's 'Passing On' revisited. *The Sociological Quarterly*, 39 (3): 453–472.

Timmermans, S (2005) Death brokering: constructing culturally appropriate deaths. *Sociology of Health and Illness*, 27 (7): 993–1013.

Timmermans, S (2007) *Postmortem: How Medical Practitioners Explain Suspicious Deaths*, 2nd edn. Chicago, IL: University of Chicago Press.

Tornstam, L (1997) Gerotranscendence: the contemplative dimension of aging. *Journal of Aging Studies*, 11 (2): 143–154.

Townsend, P (1988) *Inequalities in Health (The Black Report)*. Harmondsworth: Penguin.

Tran, M (2009) Government drug adviser David Nutt sacked. *The Guardian* 30 October. Available online at: www.guardian.co.uk/politics/2009/oct/30/drugs-adviser-david-nutt-sacked

Transform (2004) *After the War on Drugs: Options for Control*. Available online at: www.tdpf.org.uk/Transform_After_the_War_on_Drugs.pdf

Transforming Care and Commissioning Steering Group (2014) *Winterbourne View: Time for Change*. Redditch: NHS England.

Travis, A (2009) Government criticised over refusal to downgrade ecstasy. *The Guardian* 11 February. Available online at: www.guardian.co.uk/politics/2009/feb/11/ecstasy-downgrade-drugs-class

Traynor, M (2014) Caring after Francis: moral failure in nursing reconsidered. *Journal of Research in Nursing*, 19 (7–8): 546–556.

Tuckman, B (1965) Developmental sequence in small groups. *Psychological Bulletin*, 63: 384–399.

Tuckman, B and Jensen, M (1977) Stages of small-group development revisited. *Group Organization Management*, 2: 419–427.

Tuominen, R, Stolt, M and Salminen, L (2014) Social media in nursing education: the view of students. *Education Research International*, article ID 929245. Available online at: http://dx.doi.org/10.1155/2014/929245

UKCC (1986) *Project 2000: A New Preparation for Practice*. London: UKCC.

Ulrich, RS (1984) View through a window may influence recovery from surgery. *Science*, 224: 420–421.

United Nations (2012) *Millennium Development Goals*, www.un.org/millenniumgoals

Upton, J, Fletcher, M, Madoc-Sutton, H, Sheikh, A, Caress, A and Walker, S (2011) Shared decision making or paternalism in nursing consultations? A qualitative study of primary care asthma nurses' views on sharing decisions with patients regarding inhaler device selection. *Health Expectations*. Available online at: http://www.educationforhealth.org/resources.php/138

Vienna Declaration (2010) Available online at: www.viennadeclaration.com

Walker, JA, Payne, S, Jarrett, J and Ley, T (2012) *Psychology for Nurses and the Caring Professions*. Maidenhead: McGraw-Hill.

Wanless, D (2003) *Securing Good Health for the Whole Population: Population Health Trends*. HM Treasury. London: HMSO.

Webb, C (1995) Rediscovering the unpopular patient. *Journal of Advanced Nursing*, 21 (3): 466–475.

Weber, M (1992) *The Protestant Ethic and the Spirit of Capitalism*. London: Routledge (originally published in 1905 in *Archives for Social Science and Social Welfare* 20 and 21).

Welshman, J and Walmsley, J (eds) (2006) *Community Care in Perspective: Care, Control and Citizenship*. Basingstoke: Palgrave Macmillan.

Wenger, E (2000) Communities of practice: the structure of knowledge stewarding. In: Despres, C and Chauvel, D (eds) *Knowledge Horizons: The Present and the Promise of Knowledge Management*. Woburn, MA: Butterworth Heinemann.

Werb, D, Rowell, G and Guyatt, G (2010) *Effect of Drug Law Enforcement on Drug Related Violence: Evidence from a Scientific Review*. Vancouver: International Centre for Science in Drug Policy, pp. 87–94. Available online at: www.icsdp.org/docs/ICSDP-1%20-%20FINAL.pdf

Westen, D (2002) *Psychology: Brain, Behavior and Culture*. Chichester: Wiley.

Wilkinson, R and Pickett, K (2010) *The Spirit Level: Why More Equal Societies Always Do Better*. Harmondsworth: Penguin.

Willetts, G and Clarke, D (2014) Constructing nurses' professional identity through social identity theory. *International Journal of Nursing Practice*, 20 (2): 164–169.

Williams, S, Martin, P and Gabe, J (2011) The pharmaceuticalisation of society? A framework for analysis. *Sociology of Health and Illness*, 33: 710–725.

Williamson, G, Jenkinson, T and Proctor-Childs, T (2010) *Contexts of Contemporary Nursing*, 2nd edn. Exeter: Learning Matters.

Willis Commission (2012) *Quality with Compassion: The Future of Nursing Education*. Available online at: http://www.williscommission.org.uk

Wittenberg-Lyles, E, Gee, G, Oliver, D and Demires, G (2009) What patients and families don't hear: backstage communication in hospice interdisciplinary team meetings. *Journal of Housing for the Elderly*, 23: 92–105.

Wolfensberger, W (1992) *A Brief Introduction to Social Role Valorization as a High-Order Concept for Structuring Human Services*, 2nd (revised) edn. Syracuse, NY: Syracuse University Training Institute for Human Service Planning, Leadership, & Change Agentry.

Wolfensberger, W (1995) *The SRV Training Package*. Unpublished manuscript. Available online at: www.socialrolevalorization.com/articles/overview-of-srv-theory.html

Wood, E (2010) Evidence based policy for illicit drugs. *British Medical Journal*, 341 (3374).

World Business Council for Sustainable Development (WBCSD) (2011) *Vision 2050*. Available online at: www.wbcsd.org/vision2050.aspx

World Health Organization (2008) (WHO) *Closing the Gap in a Generation: Health Equity Through Action on the Social Determinants of Health*. Geneva: WHO. Available online at: http://whqlibdoc.who.int/hq/2008/WHO_IER_CSDH_08.1_eng.pdf

World Health Organization (2014) *United Nations Agencies Report Steady Progress in Saving Mothers' Lives*. Available online at: http://www.who.int/mediacentre/news/releases/2014/maternal-mortality/en

World Health Organization (2015) *International Classification of Diseases*. Available online at: http://www.who.int/classifications/icd/en

Worldwatch Institute (2010) *State of the World: Transforming Cultures from Consumerism to Sustainability*. London: Earthscan.

Wright Mills, C (1959) *The Sociological Imagination*, 40th edn. Oxford: Oxford University Press.

Wuest, J (1993) Professionalism and the evolution of nursing as a discipline: a feminist perspective. *Journal of Professional Nursing*, 10 (6): 357–367.

Yalom, I (2008) *Staring into the Sun*. London: Piatkus.

Yeung, K and Martin, J (2003) The looking glass self: an empirical test and elaboration. *Social Forces*, 81 (3): 843–879.

Zimbardo, P (2004) A situationist perspective on the psychology of evil. In: Miller, A (ed.) *The Social Psychology of Good and Evil*. New York: Guilford.

Zimbardo, P (2007) *The Lucifer Effect: Understanding How Good People Turn Evil*. New York: Random House.

Zimmerman, C (2007) Death denial: obstacle or treatment instrument for palliative care? An analysis of clinical literature. *Sociology of Health and Illness*, 29 (2): 297–314.

Zinberg, N (1984) *Drug, Set and Setting: The Basis for Controlled Intoxicant Use*. New Haven, CT: Yale University Press.

Index